Hands on Refle...

A Complete Guide

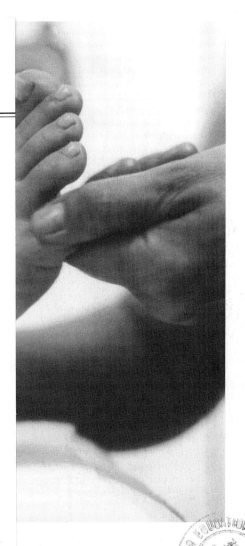

...ES

Hodder & Stoughton

A MEMBER OF THE HODDER HEADLINE GROUP

Orders: please contact Bookpoint Ltd, 130 Milton Park, Abingdon, Oxon OX14 4SB.
Telephone: (44) 01235 827720. Fax: (44) 01235 400454.
Lines are open from 9.00 – 6.00, Monday to Saturday, with a 24 hour message answering service.
You can also order through our website www.madaboutbooks.co.uk.

British Library Cataloguing in Publication Data
A catalogue record for this title is available from the British Library

ISBN 0 340 803975

First Published 2002

Impression number   10 9 8 7 6 5 4 3 2 1
Year   2007 2006 2005 2004 2003 2002

Typeset by Servis Filmsetting Ltd, Manchester
Printed in Great Britain for Hodder & Stoughton Educational, a division of Hodder Headline Plc,
338 Euston Road, London NW1 3BH by Canale Ltd.

AUTHOR FOREWORD

With love and thanks to Andrew Carter a.k.a 'Drew', without whom this book would have never left my head and reached paper!

With special love to my family and love and thanks to Nicola Jenkins for her help, support and encouragement.

With appreciation to the Association of Reflexologists for their help, support and advice throughout my reflexology career and for allowing the use of their reflexology charts.

The foot reflex chart on pages two and three is reproduced with permission by the Association of Reflexologists.

Andrew James M.A.R.

FOREWORDS

Hands on Reflexology: A Complete Guide covers the many complex facets of learning the art of reflexology. The content and layout is presented in a format suitable for use as a textbook by any student of reflexology. The clear photographs demonstrating techniques accompanying the foot and hand reflexology sequence, along with study components on reflexology, integrated biology and practice management provide a valuable reference tool.

Andrew has managed to capture the essence of the therapy in a manner which is easily understandable, and yet provides an in depth insight into the art and science that is reflexology.

Association of Reflexologists

Reflexology has proved itself to be an invaluable modality in modern health care. Andrew James, with 15 years experience as a highly successful teacher and practitioner, is well qualified to express its attributes, in this clearly written and beautifully illustrated book. I consider this essential reading for anybody interested or involved in the growing field of Integrative Health.

Christine Page MD; Author and Lecturer in Holistic Health

CONTENTS

Contents

v

vi

Contents

INTRODUCTION

Balance and wholeness are all most of us want from life. We can get lost in our everyday existence; doing more 'things' and taking on more responsibility, and thus lose sight of our own 'self'. This is when reflexology steps in. Reflexology is one of the most accessible complementary therapies; hands and feet are all you need to bring health, happiness, fun and rejuvenation to your whole being.

I have introduced reflexology to thousands of people, through individual treatment, lectures, TV and radio, conferences or talks to international companies and small self-help groups. I am still amazed that even with just a one-day workshop it is possible to see an instant change in people's physical, mental and emotional state. They leave at the end of the day feeling more balanced, literally walking on air, with something achieved for themselves; a skill that they can take home and use.

Whether you are a teacher of reflexology, a one-day workshop enthusiast, a self-starter intending to learn reflexology for the benefit of friends and family, or a student on an introductory or professional course a good, comprehensive reflexology book is an essential study aid. I have written this book with all levels in mind. I know many reflexology students may be returning to study after a long period of time so I have kept everything as straightforward and as organised as possible.

I also understand that it is difficult to know what to expect from a good reflexology book, so I have tried to take the experience of my lecturing and examining work and combine it with the comments and expectations of my students. The end result is detailed, simple and with lots of things to keep the brain active!

I hope that by splitting each area of reflexology into short, manageable chapters, with straightforward language I have made it detailed and simple and by including as many exam-type questions as possible within each chapter I have made it 'brain activated'!

I hope you will enjoy using this book – work through it from cover to cover or dip in and out of the chapters as needed. Most of all I hope it will serve you well, becoming tattered and worn – converting you, like me, into a reflexology fanatic.

Let hard work and enlightenment be the touchstone to further achievements; and may all 'the feet' you treat benefit from your continued care and understanding.

Andrew James M.A.R.

CHAPTER 1

Foot reflexology sequence (illustrated guide)

The most confusing aspect of learning the reflexology sequence is the variety of charts and diagrams available, many of which seem to vary in their depiction of the location of some reflex points. Treatment recommendations will also vary greatly. This is discussed in more detail in Chapter 6.

The following is a suggested sequence only. It is based on the reflexology chart shown in Figure 1. It is not the only possible sequence, or the only reflexology chart available. If you would prefer to use a different sequence or chart, then the following guide can still be useful as a reference point for commonly worked reflex areas. An entire treatment should last approximately 50 minutes.

BEFORE TREATMENT:

- Examine the legs and feet for varicose veins (no pressure to be applied directly over a varicose vein), verrucas (cover with plaster), athlete's foot (wipe with mild antiseptic solution or a tea tree essential oil based product).

- Wipe the feet clean with a moistened tissue product.

- Ensure that the checks for contraindications have been completed – see Chapter 8.

TECHNIQUES AND TERMINOLOGY USED IN THE SEQUENCE:

- 'Between 3/4, 1/2' or 'on zone 3' – refers to the imaginary lines that run straight down the foot between each toe, known as the longitudinal zones. See Chapter 6 for more details.

- **Hooking technique** – a direct pressure to a reflex with the side or flat of the thumb or finger. The movement and pressure are obtained by bending the thumb or finger and rotating into the appropriate reflex area.

- **Medial** – refers to the imaginary line that runs exactly down the centre of the body. So the medial side of the big toe will be the side that is nearest to the middle line of the body.

- **Lateral** – refers to the point furthest away from the imaginary line that runs exactly down the centre of the body. So the lateral side of the big toe will be the side that is furthest away from the middle line of the body.

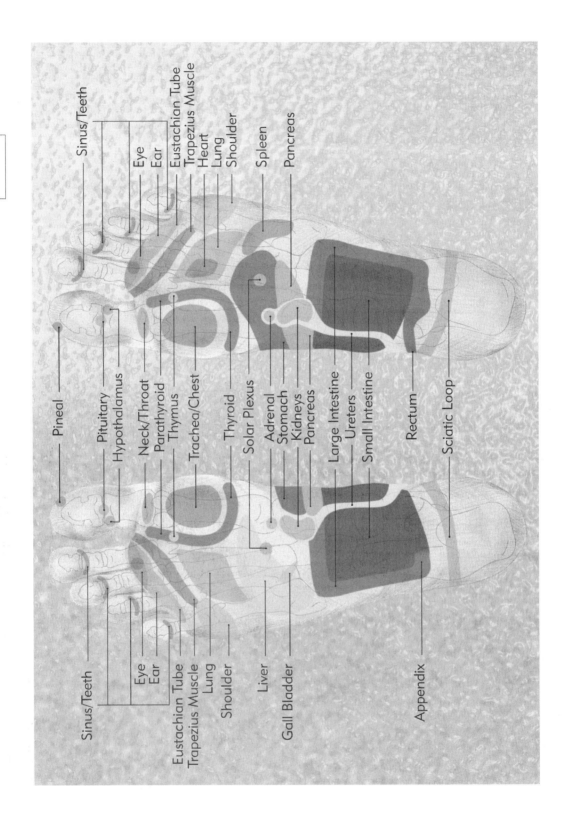

Sinus/Teeth

Eye
Ear
Eustachian Tube
Trapezius Muscle
Heart
Lung
Shoulder

Spleen

Pancreas

Pineal

Pituitary
Hypothalamus

Neck/Throat
Parathyroid
Thymus

Trachea/Chest

Thyroid

Solar Plexus

Adrenal
Stomach
Kidneys
Pancreas

Large Intestine
Ureters
Small Intestine

Rectum

Sciatic Loop

Sinus/Teeth

Eye
Ear

Eustachian Tube
Trapezius Muscle
Lung

Shoulder

Liver

Gall Bladder

Appendix

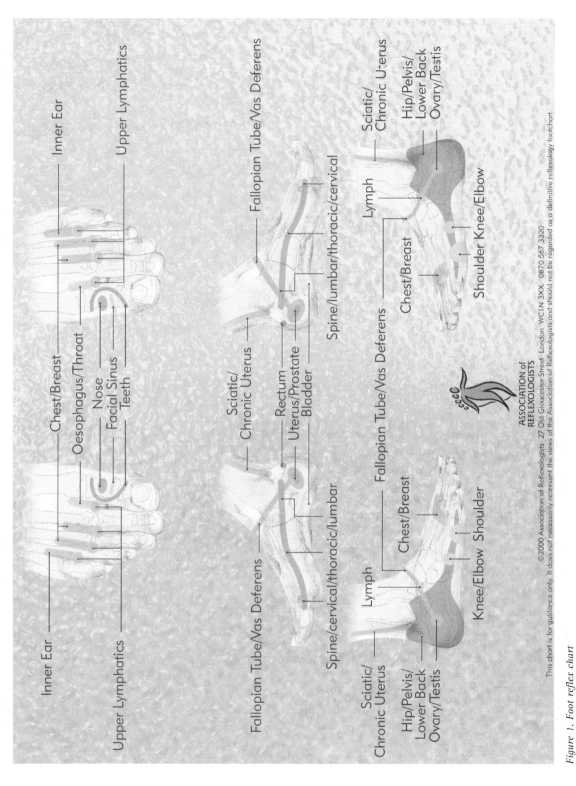

Figure 1. *Foot reflex chart*

Foot reflexology sequence (illustrated guide)

Chapter 1

- **Bites** – crawling movement with pressure of the thumb or fingers. Each movement is known as a 'bite'.

- **Rotate** – clockwise and anticlockwise movements with pressure, applied several times.

- **Press** – a steady, even pressure on a particular area.

Please note that every foot is a different size and shape and therefore any measurements given for reflex locations are approximate. Refer to the illustrations for precise locations.

THE SEQUENCE

This sequence is available on a training video by the author, visit: www.handsonreflexology.com for details.

THE OPENING MOVEMENTS

The reflex points are shown in a suggested order. Do not worry if you prefer a different order. The guide will still be useful for the location of the major reflex points.

1. **Rotate the foot**

   Take the right foot into the left hand, and hold the heel firmly. Grip the metatarsal arch with the right hand and rotate clockwise and anticlockwise several times.

   Feels relaxing to the client; helps the client get used to having their foot worked.

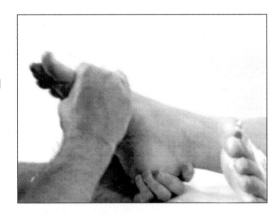

2. **Stretch the achilles**

   With the hands in the same position, stretch and relax the leg (pull the heel with the left hand).

   Relaxes the foot, helps relieve tension.

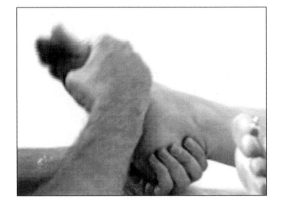

3. **Open and stretch the chest**

   Place the fingers on top of the foot so that the fingertips meet at zone 3, thumbs underneath on the metatarsal arch. Pull outwards with a gliding, pressure movement.

   Stretches the foot, helps breathing to become more regular and relaxed.

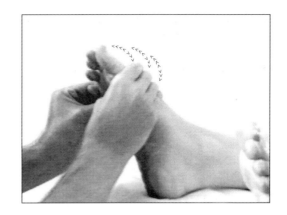

4. **Solar plexus**

   Support the foot with the left hand. Trace down on zone 2 with the right thumb to the diaphragm. Place the right thumb just below the diaphragm and press and release, then rotate.

   A plexus is a gathering of nerve endings. The solar plexus is often called the brain of the abdomen; it receives signals from the brain and transmits them to the organs of the abdomen.

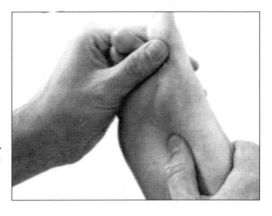

Repeat movements 1–4 on the left foot (reversing hand positions i.e. left thumb for left solar plexus) – *then return to the right foot.*

5. **Cervical vertebrae**

   Sandwich the foot with the left hand. With the right thumb work up towards the big toe with seven bites (repeat three times).

   The seven smallest bones of the spine, the cervical vertebrae gives the head its movement and supports the skull.

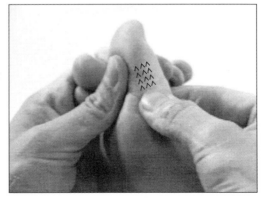

Foot reflexology sequence (illustrated guide)

Chapter 1

5

6. Head and neck

Support the toes of the right foot with the left hand. Place the right hand over the left hand. Place the right thumb on the medial side of the big toe. Work over the big toe with bites down to the lateral base of the big toe. Then repeat.

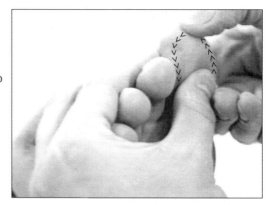

7. Brain

With the medial side of the right thumb, work over the brain on top of the big toe with bites in three rows, slightly lower with each row.

The centre of control for the whole body, the right side of the brain controls the left side of the body, and the left side of the brain controls the right side of the body. The brain deals with vast amounts of information, processing our external view of the world and is the control hub for many conscious and unconscious bodily functions. It is also the centre for our thoughts and emotions and many of its complex functions governing our feelings of 'self' are still undiscovered.

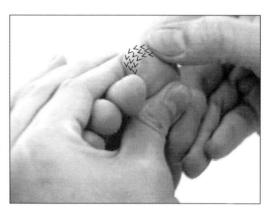

8. Front of neck

Support the top of the big toe with left hand. Make a 'bird's beak' with the thumb and the first and second finger of the right hand. Place at the base of the big toe on the medial side. With the first and second fingers work around the front of the big toe with bites, in rows, working higher with each row until you reach the base of the toenail.

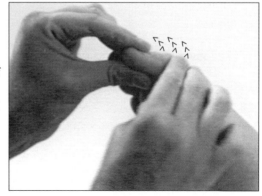

The first row will also treat the throat area; the higher rows will treat the lower and upper jaw.

9. **Back of neck**

   Hold the same fingers to support the front of the big toe. With the right thumb work the back of the big toe, taking bites medial to lateral in three rows, each row lower than the other, until you reach the base of the big toe.

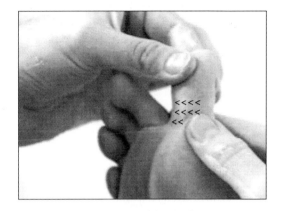

10. **Occipital**

    From the finishing place of the back of the neck (above) work up three bites to the Occipital (on the lateral side of the big toe). Rotate.

    A bone forming the rear and rear bottom of the skull.

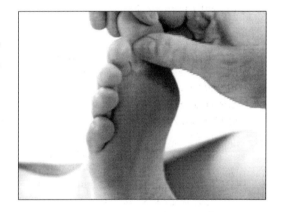

11. **Ear**

    From the Occipital point continue upward three more bites to the ear. Rotate.

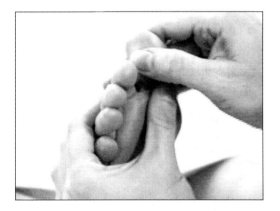

12. Hypothalamus

Slide the right thumb across to the medial side of the big toe and rotate.

Part of the endocrine system, this acts as a link between the pituitary and the brain. It controls the autonomic nervous system and regulates body heat.

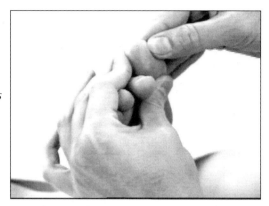

13. Pineal

This worked at the same time as the hypothalamus (above).

A gland that forms part of the endocrine system. It secretes melatonin and controls the rhythms of the body such as sleeping and waking.

14. Pituitary

With the right thumb, rotate to the lateral side of the centre point of the big toe (this feels like a little pea to the client). If difficult to locate then bend the index finger and use the knuckle to rotate the point.

The 'master' gland of the endocrine system, controlling all other endocrine glands so that they function in harmony.

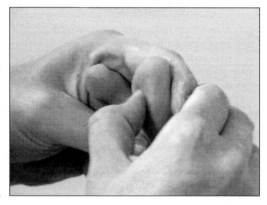

15. Sinuses

Support the second toe with the left hand. With the right thumb take bites up the medial side until you reach the top. Change positions to support the toe with the right hand and with the left thumb take bites up the lateral side until you reach the top. Then take bites from the base of the back of the toe upwards, until just before the top. Slide with pressure over the top of the toe to help drain the sinuses. Repeat for each toe.

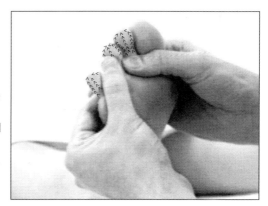

Sinuses are hollow cavities within the bone structure of the face. Lined with hair and mucous membrane, they form a defence against dust, germs etc. Blocked sinuses cause pain.

16. General eye and ear

Place the left thumb at the back of the foot, below the base of the toes, with the rest of the hand resting on the front of the foot. Now stretch down lightly to open the padded area at the base of the toes at the back. Work on the padded area under all the toes with bites, using the right thumb from medial to lateral, and then reverse hand positions to work back again with the left thumb from lateral to medial.

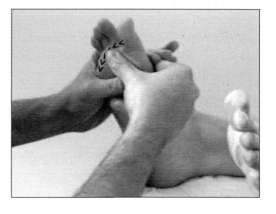

A helper area to the specific eye and ear points.

17. Eye

With the right thumb press the point under the toes between 2/3.

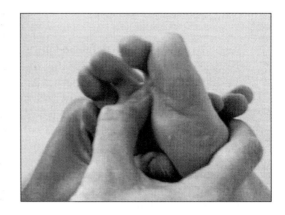

18. Ear

With the right thumb press the point under the toes between 4/5.

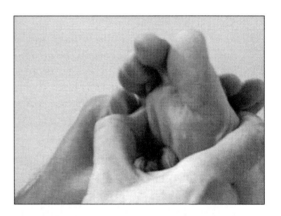

19. Eustachian tube

Support the foot with the right hand and with the left index finger and thumb take bites down between 3/4 for about 1 cm. Then take bites back up until between the toes. Press and rotate between 3/4.

This is a tube that runs from the middle ear to the top of the throat/back of the nose.

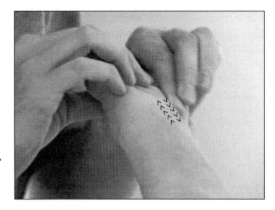

20. Balance

Press the front of the base of the fourth toe with the left-hand index finger on top and the thumb supporting underneath.

Helps with inner ear and balance problems.

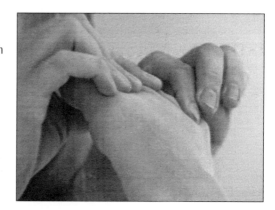

21. Shoulder

With the left hand (index finger on top and thumb underneath foot) work with bites down about 5 cm between 4/5 then work up and down this area with bites and pressure.

Trace down the sole about 3.5 cm with either thumb on zone 4 underneath the foot. Take bites up to the base of the toes; repeat this in upward rows from medial to lateral until the outer edge of zone 5.

A ball and socket joint connecting the arm to the trunk of the body.

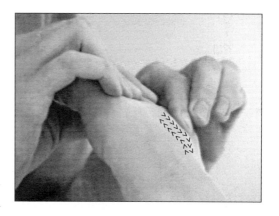

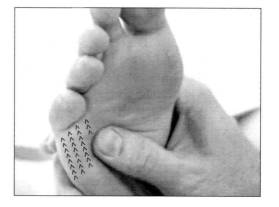

22. Diaphragm

Support the top of the foot with the left hand. Work the diaphragm with the right thumb with bites from medial to lateral and then reverse the hand positions to work with the left thumb from lateral to medial (half-moon shape).

A muscular dome-shaped membrane dividing the chest cavity from the abdomen. It helps control the filling and emptying of the lungs.

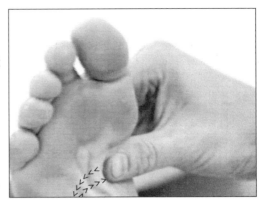

23. Thyroid

Support the foot with the left hand. With the right thumb start at the diaphragm (22) and work three to four rows upwards with bites up to the base of the big toe, working from lateral to medial.

On the last row turn the thumb to work across the same area, medial to lateral; work down for each row, finishing at the diaphragm line.

An endocrine gland with two lobes that regulates the body's metabolic rate and secretes thyroxin.

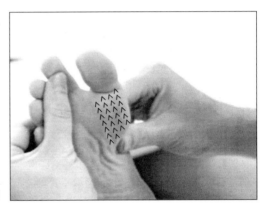

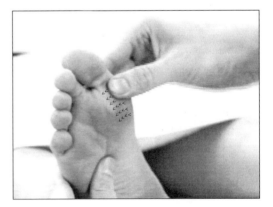

24. Parathyroid

Support the foot with the right hand. With the left index finger and thumb press between the toes of 1 and 2 and then rotate.

Four small endocrine glands found behind each side of the thyroid. Controls phosphorous and calcium levels.

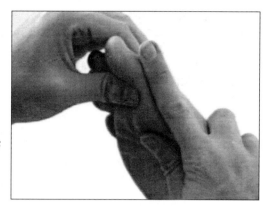

25. Thymus

Support the foot with the right hand. With the left hand come down to halfway between the parathyroid and diaphragm. Hook in, then press and rotate.

A gland in which lymphocytes mature and multiply. Lymphocytes help the body to fight infection.

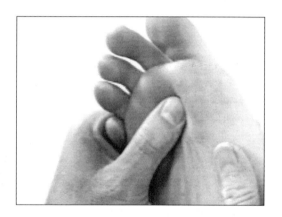

26. Lungs

Hold back the toes gently with the left hand. With the right thumb work up with bites from the diaphragm between zones 2/3, 3/4, 4/5.

The lungs are the principal organs of the respiratory system; they take in oxygen and expel carbon dioxide.

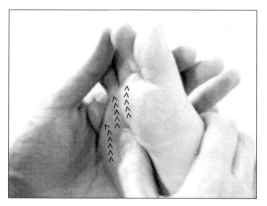

27. Gall bladder

Hold the foot with the left hand. Trace down zone 3. Press in approximately 1 cm under the diaphragm with the right thumb towards the little toe. Rotate.

Stores and concentrates bile from the liver, ready to release into the intestine. Bile helps break down fats so that they can be absorbed by the body.

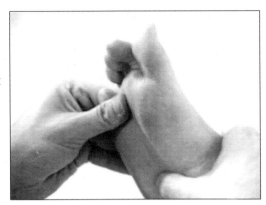

28. Liver

From the gall bladder work three rows in bites from medial to lateral into the fifth zone, working slightly lower with each row. Repeat the rows using the left thumb and taking bites from lateral to medial back to the gall bladder.

Produces bile, vitamins and minerals. Filters waste products and produces blood-clotting compounds. It is the main organ of detoxification.

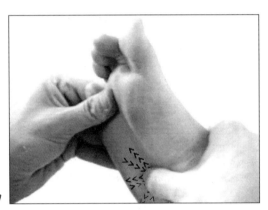

29. Stomach/pancreas

Sandwich the foot with the left hand. Place the right thumb under the diaphragm on zone 1. Work with the right thumb from medial to lateral until zone 3, moving downwards with three rows.

Main organ of digestion. Breaks down food with gastric juices.

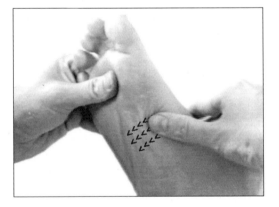

30. Duodenum and small intestine

Stop at the end of the third row (29); rotate and work down in bites and rotations towards the heel for the duodenum and part of the small intestine.

The intestine is the largest organ of the digestive system. Food is moved through it by peristalsis (wavelike contractions).

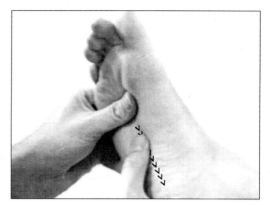

31. Ileo-caecal valve (ICV) and colon

Place the left thumb on the ICV approximately 5 cm from the heel between zones 4 and 5, then press and rotate. Use the thumb to work up in bites, following ascending colon to hepatic flexure. Hook in and rotate. Lift the elbow and swivel the thumb to work in bites across the transverse colon from lateral to medial, ending at zone 1.

The ICV is a one-way valve that opens into the colon. The colon is also known as the large intestine. It holds waste products until they are emptied through the anus.

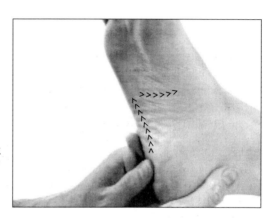

32. Small intestine/colon helper area

Hold the foot with the right hand. Lift the left thumb and place just below the transverse colon on zone 4. Take bites across to zone 1. Repeat for three or four rows, with each row lower than the previous.

The intestine is the largest organ of the digestive system. Food is moved through it by peristalsis (wavelike contractions).

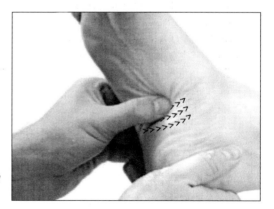

33. Lower back/colon helper area

Support the foot with the left hand. With the right hand (side of hand/pad of thumb) use light massage rotation movements down the medial side of the leg from the knee to the ankle. Place the side of the hand/pad of the thumb on the heel area and stretch medially.

Can help with chronic lower back pain, haemorrhoids and constipation.

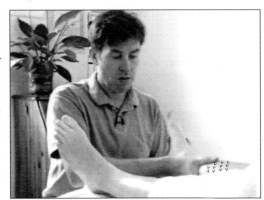

34. Uterus (female)/prostate (male)

Sandwich the foot with the left hand. Find the point on the medial side of the foot that is approximately halfway between the ankle and the heel. Press and rotate with the right thumb.

Part of the male and female reproductive systems. For females, work lightly if first or second day of menstruation.

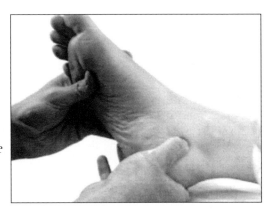

35. Ovary (female)/testes (male)

Sandwich the foot with the right hand. Find the point on the lateral side of the foot that is approximately halfway between the ankle and the heel. Press and rotate with the left thumb.

Endocrine glands form part of the male and female reproductive system.

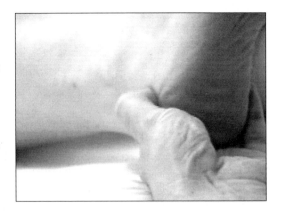

36. Fallopian tubes (female)/vas deferens (male)

With the left thumb work in bites over the top of the foot, lateral to medial to link from ovary/testes/to uterus/prostate.

Part of the male and female reproductive systems

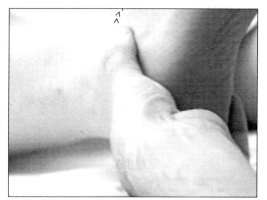

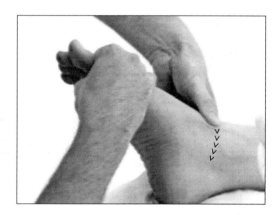

37. Lymphatics

From the position above, with the index and second finger of the right hand take bites from medial to lateral, working slightly higher than previously until you reach the testes/ovary area.

With the left thumb work in bites to cover three semicircular rows around the lateral ankle. The first row should be close to the ankle, the other rows becoming further away and larger (like ripples on a pond). Both sides (in front of and behind) the lateral ankle should be worked.

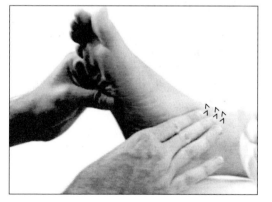

With the right thumb perform the same technique on the medial ankle.

The secondary circulation system. Protects, cleanses and helps remove waste products from the body.

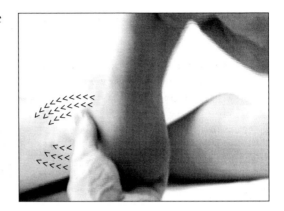

38. Sciatic nerve

From the last row of the medial ankle work down with the right thumb in bites towards the heel. Press the sciatic point just before the heel. Continue working down with bites until you reach the sole of the foot.

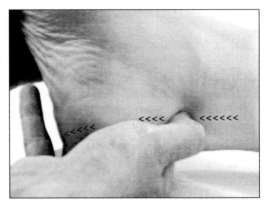

Continue with bites, working across the sole of the foot via the sciatic loop from medial to lateral. When you reach the lateral side of the sole change thumbs and work in bites up the heel towards the sciatic point on the lateral side. Press and rotate the sciatic point with the left thumb – this should be the same level as the medial sciatic point.

The strongest and largest nerve of the body. Runs from the lumbar region to branch down the back of each leg.

39. Shoulder, upper arm, elbow, lower arm, wrist

Sandwich the foot with the right hand then place the left thumb below the small toe on zone 5. Work down the side of the foot with bites up to the bony prominence.

The shoulder is a ball and socket joint; the elbow is a hinge joint and the wrist is a gliding joint.

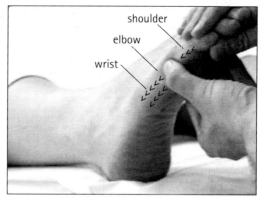

40. Knee, hip, lower back

Using the left thumb lift over the bony prominence then rotate into the area for the knee point. Take bites to reach the hip point then rotate; take more bites to reach the lower back then rotate.

The knee is a hinge joint and the hip is a ball and socket joint.

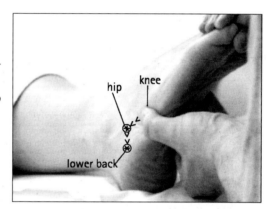

41. Chronic back helper area/lower back/sacro-iliac joint and pelvis

Taking bites with the left thumb, work from the lower back point towards the back of the heel; work in rows, each row above the previous until the heel area is worked.

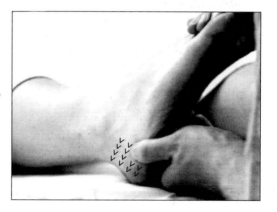

Repeat the action with the right thumb on the medial side, with each row lower than the last until you finish on the coccyx point. Press and rotate the coccyx point.

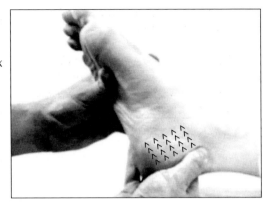

42. Bladder

With the right thumb on the coccyx, work bites in four to five rows, following the fan-shaped, puffy, softer area.

A muscular sack that holds urine until it is passed out of the body.

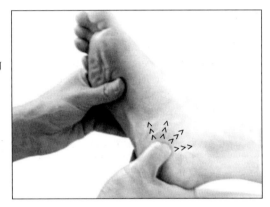

43. Ureter and kidney

Continue with the right thumb. Take three bites laterally from the centre of the bladder to the start of the ureter.

With the right thumb take bites to work up the ureter (in the direction of the toes) to the kidney point.

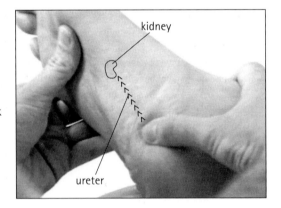

kidney

ureter

Rotate, press, then trigger the kidney point with the right thumb.

The ureter is a muscular tube that extends from the kidney to the bladder. The kidney collects and filters toxins, salts and other waste products.

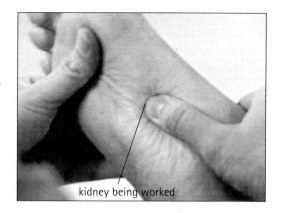

kidney being worked

44. Adrenals

Take the left hand away from the supporting position then hook in, lift, press and rotate the adrenal point directly above the kidney with the left thumb (light pressure).

Small endocrine glands that secrete adrenaline, hydrocortisones and other substances.

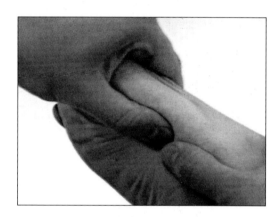

45. Cervical spine

Sandwich the foot with the left hand. With the lateral side of the right thumb take seven bites downwards, pressing with each bite. Repeat.

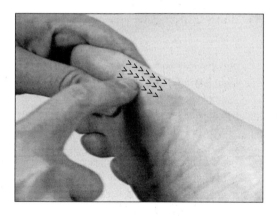

46. Thoracic spine – downwards

Slide over the joint and continue in a downwards movement with 12 bites, pressing after each bite.

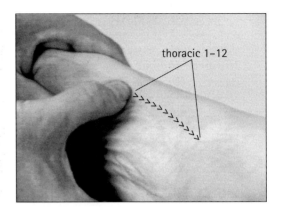

thoracic 1–12

47. Lumbar spine – downwards

Continue in a downwards movement with five bites (slightly higher on the arch of the foot), pressing after each bite.

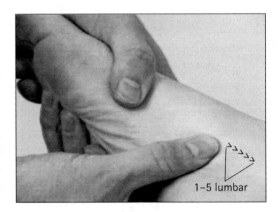

1–5 lumbar

48. Coccyx/lower back and sciatic helper area

After the fifth lumbar point, replace the right thumb with the left thumb or index finger (as an anchor point). Using the right thumb, rotate the coccyx point. From the coccyx point work in bites down towards the heel, turning to work upwards towards the sciatic area. When the thumb is parallel to the anchor point, turn and work towards it. The right thumb will then meet the anchor point. Remove the anchor point and replace it with the right thumb, preparing to work back up the spine.

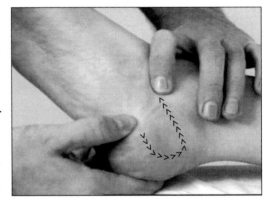

49. Lumbar spine – upwards

With the right thumb work five bites upwards (in the direction of the big toe), pressing after each bite.

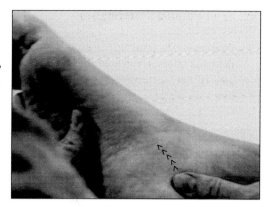

50. Thoracic spine – upwards

Continue in an upwards movement, with 12 bites, pressing after each bite.

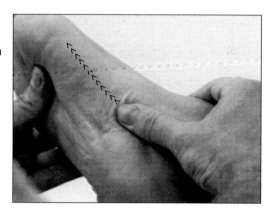

51. Thoracic spine – downwards

Turn the right thumb to face in a downwards direction (towards the heel) and repeat the 12 bites.

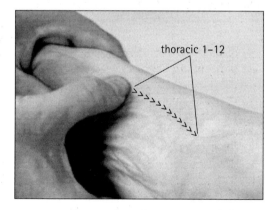

thoracic 1–12

52. Lumbar spine – downwards

Continue in a downwards movement with five bites (slightly higher on the arch of the foot), pressing after each bite.

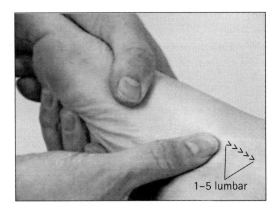

1–5 lumbar

53. Coccyx and sacral area

After the fifth lumbar point, replace the right thumb with the left thumb or index finger (as an anchor point). Using the right thumb rotate the coccyx point. From the coccyx point work in bites directly up to the anchor point. Repeat several times to cover the sacral area. Remove the anchor point and replace it with the right thumb, preparing to work back up the spine.

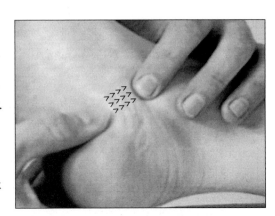

54. Lumbar spine – upwards

With the right thumb work five bites upwards (in the direction of the big toe), pressing after each bite.

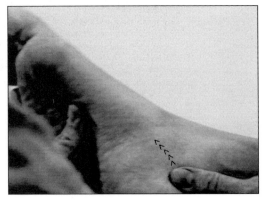

55. Thoracic spine – upwards

Continue in an upwards movement, with 12 bites, pressing after each bite.

The spine consists of vertebrae – bones with the flexibility to allow movement and protect the spinal cord (nerve pathway). In total, there are 7 cervical, 12 thoracic, 5 lumbar, 5 sacrum (fused) and 4 coccyx (fused).

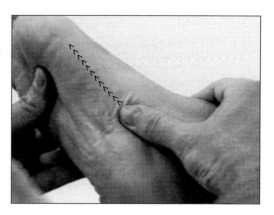

56. Spinal nerves

Repeat the 12 bites of the thoracic spine and five bites of the lumbar spine but in a sideways direction (moving downwards). Return up the spine with five bites of the lumbar and 12 bites of the thoracic, again in a sideways direction.

The spinal nerves run down the spinal column and branch off at various points to supply the major organs of the body.

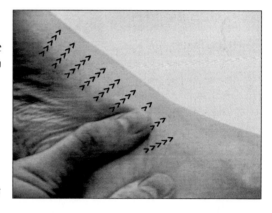

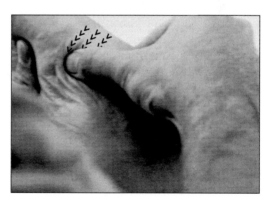

57. Lymphatic

Starting between zone 1/2, with the left index finger on top of the foot and the thumb underneath, take bites down about 5 cm between the toes. Rotate, then draw back, applying pressure with the thumb and index finger in a draining movement. Repeat between each zone.

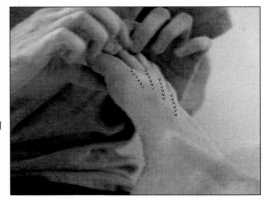

58. Chest/breast area

Using the finger pads of the left hand, take bites in two rows across the top of the foot, the second row lower than the first, from lateral to medial, across zones 5/4/3. Then glide down, applying light pressure with finger pads.

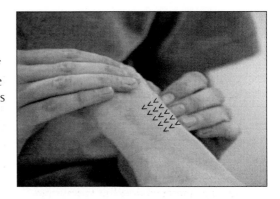

59. Open and stretch chest area

Place the fingers on top of the foot so that the fingertips meet at zone 3, with the thumbs underneath on the metatarsal arch. Pull outwards with a gliding, pressure movement.

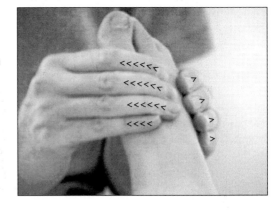

60. Energise zones

Support with the left hand. Starting at the top of the ankle with the right hand, work four or five bites across all the zones from medial to lateral; working up towards the toes with each row.

Stimulates the longitudinal zone pathways, helping with energy flow.

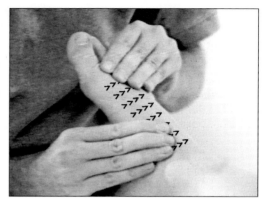

61. Rotate, stretch and drain

Support the foot with the right hand. With the left hand rotate the toes (clockwise and anticlockwise) holding them at the base, and stretch.

With the left thumb and index finger of the left hand take several bites downwards between the toes for about 5 cm. Pull back towards the toes, keeping pressure with the thumb and index finger.

Helps to further stimulate the upper lymphatic system and drain toxins.

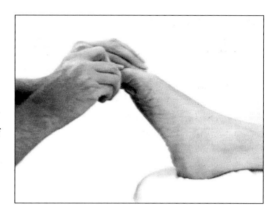

THE LEFT FOOT

62. Cervical vertebrae

Sandwich the foot with the right hand. With the left thumb work up towards the big toe with seven bites (repeat three times).

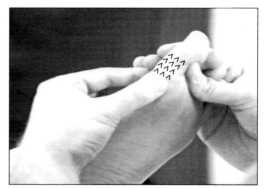

63. Head and neck

Support the toes of the left foot with
the right hand. Place the left hand
over the right hand. Place the left thumb
on the medial side of the big toe. Work
over the big toe with bites down to the
lateral base of the big toe. Then repeat.

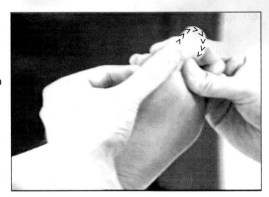

64. Brain

With the medial side of the left thumb,
work over the brain on top of the big
toe with bites in three rows, slightly
lower with each row.

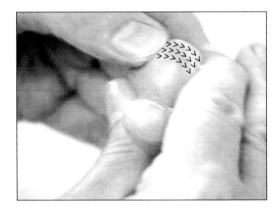

65. Front of neck

Support the top of the big toe with the
right hand. Make a 'bird's beak' with the
thumb, and the first and second finger
of the left hand. Place at the base of the
big toe on the medial side. With the first
and second fingers work around the
front of the big toe with bites, in rows,
working higher with each row until you
reach the base of the toenail.

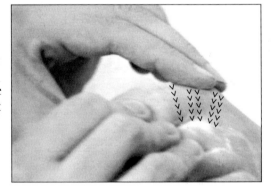

66. Back of neck

Hold the same fingers to support the front of the big toe. With the left thumb work the back of the big toe, taking bites medial to lateral in three rows, each row lower than the other, until you reach the base of the big toe.

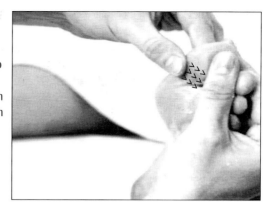

67. Occipital

From the finishing place of the back of the neck (above) work up three bites to the occipital (on the lateral side of the big toe). Rotate.

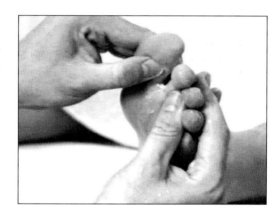

68. Ear

From the Occipital point continue upwards three more bites to the ear. Rotate.

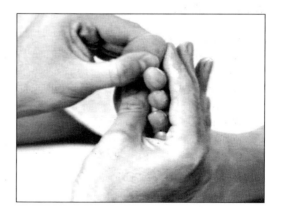

69. Hypothalamus

Slide the left thumb across to the medial side of the big toe and rotate.

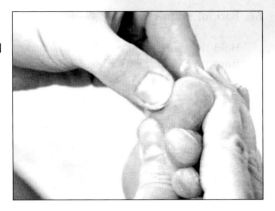

70. Pineal

This is worked at the same time as the hypothalamus (above).

71. Pituitary

With the left thumb, rotate to the lateral side of the centre point of the big toe (this feels like a little pea to the client). If difficult to locate then bend the index finger and use the knuckle to rotate the point.

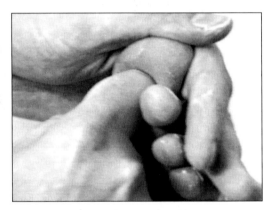

72. Sinuses

Support the second toe with the right hand. With the left thumb take bites up the medial side until you reach the top. Change positions to support the toe with the left hand, and with the right thumb take bites up the lateral side until you reach the top. Then take bites from the base of the back of the toe upwards, until just before the top. Slide with pressure over the top of the toe to help drain the sinuses. Repeat for each toe.

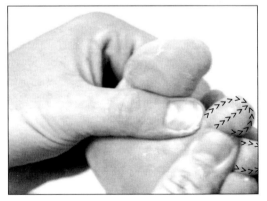

73. General eye and ear

Place the right thumb at the back of the foot, below the base of the toes, with the rest of the hand resting on the front of the foot. Now stretch down lightly to open the padded area at the base of the toes at the back. Work on the padded area under all the toes with bites, using the left thumb from medial to lateral, and then reverse hand positions to work back again with the right thumb from lateral to medial.

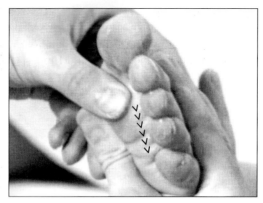

74. Eye

With the left thumb press the point under the toes between 2/3.

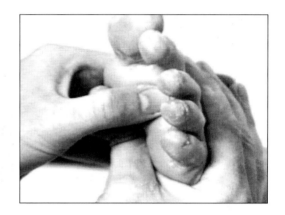

75. Ear

With the left thumb press the point under the toes between 4/5.

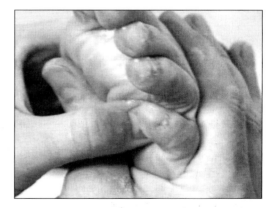

76. Eustachian tube

Support the foot with the left hand and
with the right index finger and thumb
take bites down between 3/4 for about
1 cm. Then take bites back up until
between the toes. Press and rotate
between 3/4.

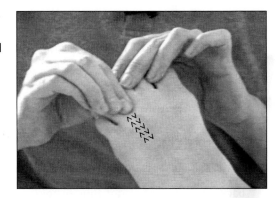

77. Balance

Press the front of the base of the fourth
toe with the right-hand index finger on
top and the thumb supporting
underneath.

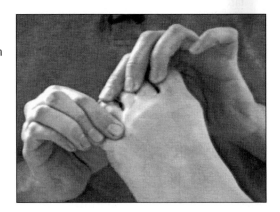

78. Shoulder

With the right hand (index finger on top
and thumb underneath foot) work with
bites down about 5 cm between 4/5
then work up and down this area with
bites and pressure.

Trace down about 3.5 cm with either
thumb on zone 4 underneath the foot.
Take bites up to the base of the toes;
repeat this in upward rows from medial
to lateral until the outer edge of zone 5.

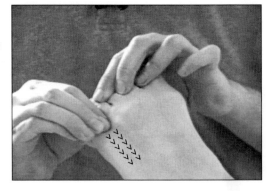

79. Diaphragm

Support the top of the foot with the right hand. Work the diaphragm with the left thumb with bites from medial to lateral and then reverse hand positions to work with the right thumb from lateral to medial (half-moon shape).

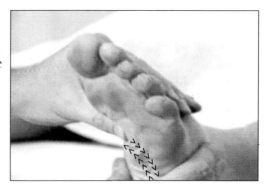

80. Thyroid

Support the foot with the right hand. With the left thumb start at the diaphragm and work three to four rows upwards with bites up to the base of the big toe, working from lateral to medial.

On the last row turn the thumb to work across the same area, medial to lateral; work down for each row, finishing at the diaphragm line.

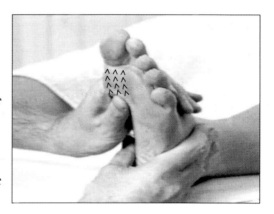

81. Parathyroid

Support the foot with the left hand. With the right index finger and thumb press between the toes of 1 and 2 and then rotate.

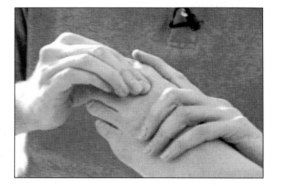

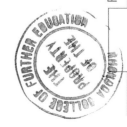

82. Thymus

Support the foot with the left hand. With the right hand come down to halfway between the parathyroid and diaphragm. Hook in, then press and rotate.

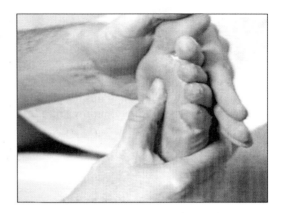

83. Lungs

Hold back the toes gently with the right hand. With the left thumb work up with bites from the diaphragm between zones 2/3, 3/4, 4/5.

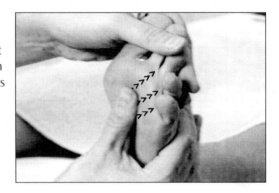

84. Cardiac area

Support the foot with the left hand. With the right thumb take bites in three rows from zone 5 to zone 1/2. The first row starts below the general eye and ear area, with each row lower than the previous until finishing just above the diaphragm line.

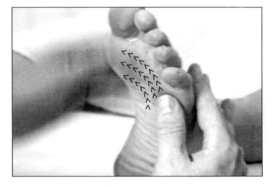

85. Heart

Moving the right thumb down on 4 to halfway between the base of the fourth toe and the diaphragm line, press the heart reflex with right thumb rotations. Then put the right index finger on top of the foot to place corresponding to the thumb. Apply pressure with index finger.

One of the strongest muscles in the body. Provides the pump to move deoxygenated blood from the veins to the lungs and oxygenated blood from the lungs to the arteries.

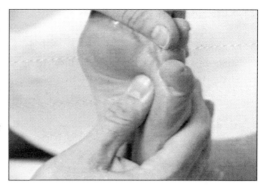

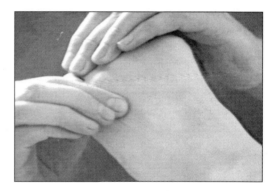

86. Spleen

Move the right thumb down between 4/5 to just under the diaphragm and rotate.

Contains lymph and blood vessels. Cleans and recycles red blood cells, filters toxins and produces lympholytes.

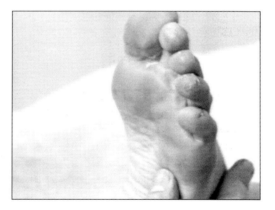

87. Stomach/pancreas

From the spleen, with the right thumb, take bites across the foot in three rows, from lateral to medial, each row lower than the other.

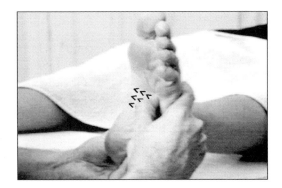

88. Transverse and descending colon

Place the left thumb underneath the finishing position of the right thumb (above) and take bites across the foot from medial to lateral. Change thumbs then rotate the splenic flexure; then take bites down the descending colon to the sigmoid flexure, and rotate.

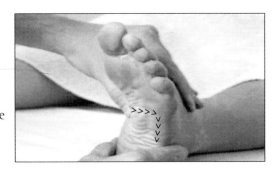

With the left thumb on the medial side of the heel, take bites towards the right thumb. Swap thumbs and take bites back towards the medial heel, along the sigmoid colon to the rectum.

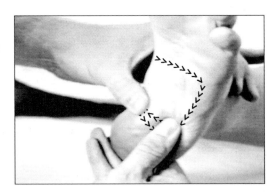

89. Small intestine/colon helper area

Hold the foot with the left hand. Lift the right thumb and place just below the transverse colon on zone 4. Take bites across to zone 1. Repeat for three or four rows, with each row lower than the previous.

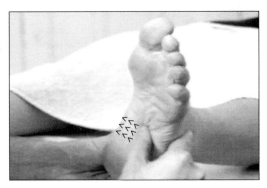

90. Lower back/colon helper area

Support the foot with the right hand. With the left hand (side of hand/pad of thumb) use light massage rotation movements down the medial side of the leg from the knee to the ankle. Place the side of the hand/pad of the thumb on the heel area and stretch medially.

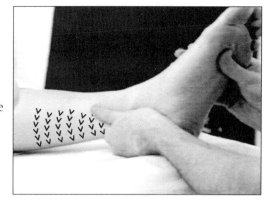

91. Uterus (female)/prostate (male)

Sandwich the foot with the right hand. Find the point on the medial side of the foot that is approximately halfway between the ankle and the heel. Press and rotate with the left thumb.

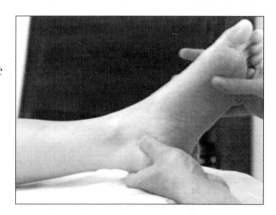

92. Ovary (female)/testes (male)

Sandwich the foot with the left hand. Find the point on the lateral side of the foot that is approximately halfway between the ankle and the heel. Press and rotate with the right thumb.

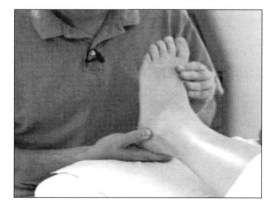

93. Fallopian tubes (female)/vas deferens (male)

With the right thumb work in bites over the top of the foot, lateral to medial, to link from ovary/testes to uterus/prostate.

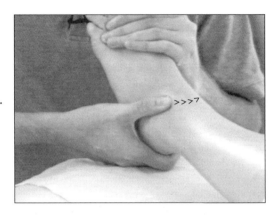

94. Lymphatics

From the position above, with the index and second finger of the left hand, take bites from medial to lateral, working slightly higher than previously until you reach the testes/ovary area.

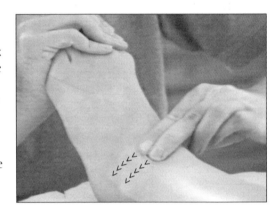

With the right thumb, work in bites to cover three semicircular rows around the lateral ankle; the first row should be close to the ankle, the other rows becoming further away and larger (like ripples on a pond). Both sides (in front of and behind) the lateral ankle should be worked.

With the left thumb perform the same technique on the medial ankle.

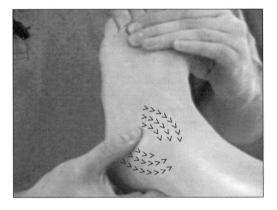

95. Sciatic nerve

From the last row of the medial ankle, work down with left thumb in bites towards the heel. Press the sciatic point just before the heel. Continue working down with bites until you reach sole of the the foot.

Continue with bites, working across the sole of the foot via the sciatic loop from medial to lateral. When you reach the lateral side of the sole, change thumbs and work in bites up the heel towards the sciatic point on the lateral side. Press and rotate the sciatic point with the right thumb – this should be the same level as the medial sciatic point.

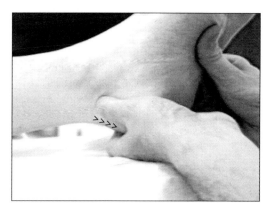

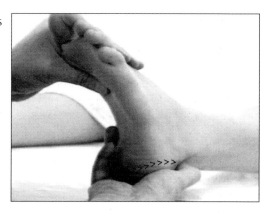

96. Shoulder, upper arm, elbow, lower arm, wrist

Sandwich the foot with the left hand then place the right thumb below the small toe on zone 5. Work down the side of the foot with bites up to the bony prominence.

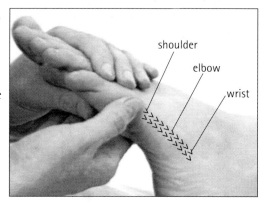

shoulder

elbow

wrist

97. Knee, hip, lower back

Using the right thumb, lift over the bony prominence then rotate into the area for the knee point. Take bites to reach the hip point then rotate; take more bites to reach the lower back then rotate.

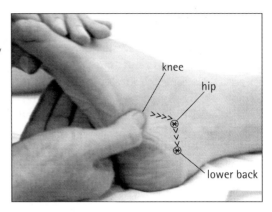

98. Chronic back helper area/lower back/sacro-iliac joint and pelvis

Taking bites with the right thumb, work from the lower back point towards the back of the heel; work in rows, each row above the previous until the heel area is worked.

Repeat the action with the left thumb on the medial side with each row lower than the last until finishing on the coccyx point.

Press and rotate the coccyx point.

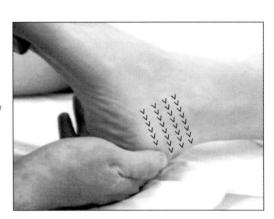

99. Bladder

With the left thumb on the coccyx, work bites in four to five rows, following the softer fan-shaped area.

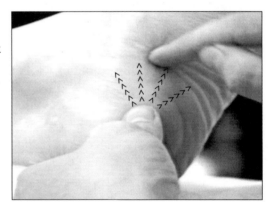

100. Ureter and kidney

Continue with the left thumb. Take three bites laterally from the centre of the bladder to the start of the ureter.

With the left thumb take bites to work up the ureter (in the direction of the toes) to the kidney point. Rotate the kidney point with the left thumb.

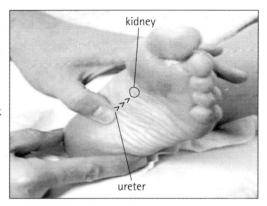

kidney

ureter

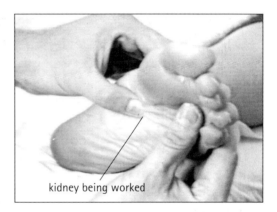

kidney being worked

101. Adrenals

Take the right hand away from the supporting position then hook in, lift, press and rotate the adrenal point directly above the kidney with the right thumb.

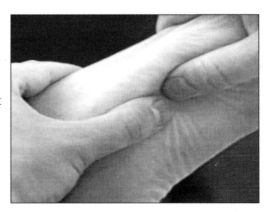

102. Cervical spine

Sandwich the foot with the right hand. With the lateral side of the left thumb take seven bites downwards, pressing with each bite. Repeat.

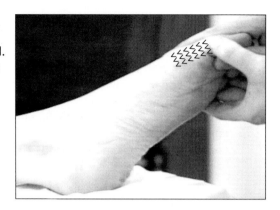

103. Thoracic spine – downwards

Continue in a downwards movement with 12 bites, pressing after each bite.

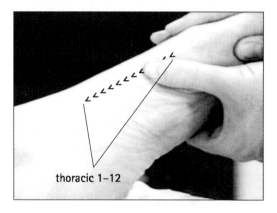

thoracic 1–12

104. Lumbar spine – downwards

Continue in a downwards movement with five bites (slightly higher on the arch of the foot), pressing after each bite.

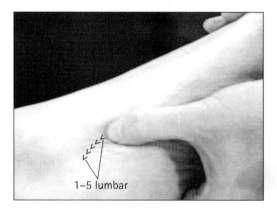

1–5 lumbar

105. Coccyx/lower back and sciatic helper area

After the fifth lumbar point, replace the left thumb with the right thumb or index finger (as an anchor point). Using the left thumb, rotate the coccyx point. From the coccyx point work in bites down towards the heel, turning to work upwards towards the sciatic area. When the thumb is parallel to the anchor point, turn and work towards it. The left thumb will then meet the anchor point. Remove the anchor point and replace it with the left thumb, preparing to work back up the spine.

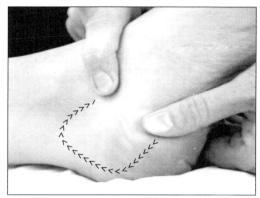

106. Lumbar spine – upwards

With the left thumb work five bites upwards (in the direction of the big toe), pressing after each bite.

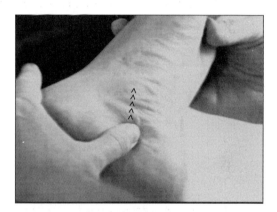

107. Thoracic spine – upwards

Continue in an upwards movement, with 12 bites, pressing after each bite.

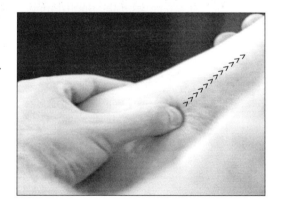

108. Thoracic spine – downwards

Turn the left thumb to face in a downwards direction (towards the heel) and using the lateral side of the thumb repeat the 12 bites.

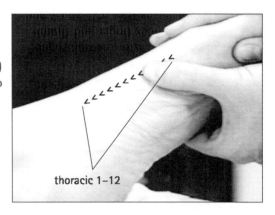

thoracic 1–12

109. Lumbar spine – downwards

Continue in a downwards movement with five bites (slightly higher on the arch of the foot), pressing after each bite.

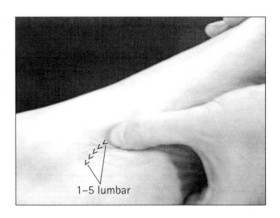

1–5 lumbar

110. Coccyx and sacral area

After the fifth lumbar point, replace the left thumb with the right thumb or index finger (as an anchor point). Using the left thumb rotate the coccyx point. From the coccyx point work in bites directly up to the anchor point. Repeat several times to cover the sacral area. Remove the anchor point and replace it with the left thumb, preparing to work back up the spine.

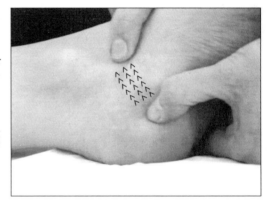

111. Lumbar spine – upwards

With the left thumb work five bites upwards (in the direction of the big toe), pressing after each bite.

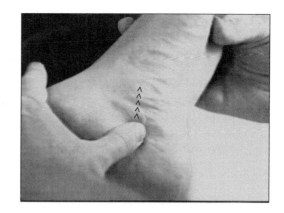

112. Thoracic spine – upwards

Continue in an upwards movement, with 12 bites, pressing after each bite.

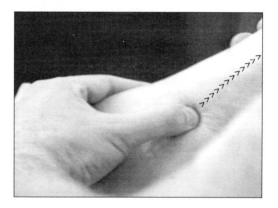

113. Spinal nerves

Repeat the 12 bites of the thoracic spine and five bites of the lumbar spine but in a sideways direction (moving downwards). Return up the spine with five bites of the lumbar and 12 bites of the thoracic, again in a sideways direction.

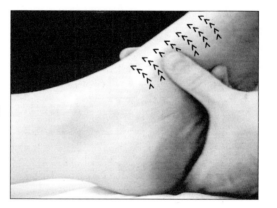

114. Lymphatic

Starting between zone 1/2, with the right index finger on top of the foot and the thumb underneath, take bites down about 5 cm between the toes. Rotate, then draw back, applying pressure with the thumb and index finger in a draining movement. Repeat between each toe.

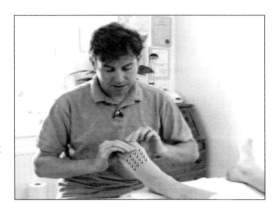

115. Chest/breast area

Using the finger pads of the right hand, take bites in two rows, the second row lower than the first, across the top of the foot, from lateral to medial, across zones 5/4/3. Then glide down, applying light pressure with finger pads.

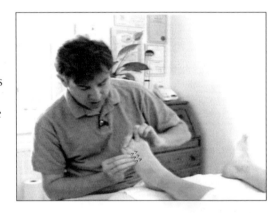

116. Open and stretch chest area

Place the fingers on top of the foot so that the fingertips meet at zone 3, with the thumbs underneath on the metatarsal arch. Pull outwards with a gliding, pressure movement.

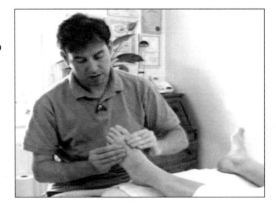

117. Energise zones

Support with right hand. Starting at top of ankle with left hand work 4 or 5 bites across all the zones from the medial to lateral. Work up towards the toes with each row.

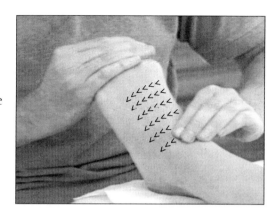

118. Rotate, stretch and drain

Support the foot with the left hand. With the right hand rotate the toes (clockwise and anticlockwise) holding them at the base, and stretch.

With the thumb and index finger of the right hand, take several bites downwards between the toes for about 5 cm. Pull back towards the toes, keeping pressure with the thumb and index finger.

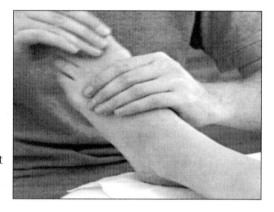

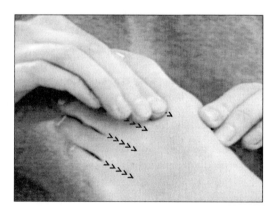

THE CLOSING MOVEMENTS

Return to the right foot.

119. Foot massage

Place both thumbs under the right foot and all fingers on top of the foot around the ankle area. Rotate the fingers in circular massage-like movements. Continue these movements, working up towards the toes. Repeat several times.

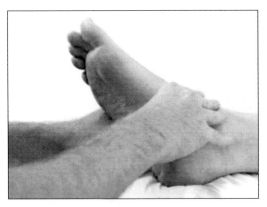

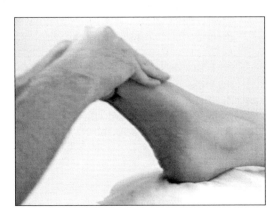

120. Spinal release

Hold the foot with both hands on the medial side, close to the ankle. Lift and pull away gently with the leading hand (the hand nearest the toes). Repeat, moving up the spine towards the toes.

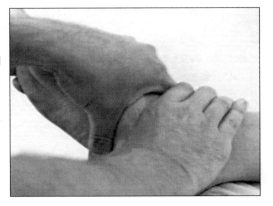

121. Chest release

Move the leading hand across to the lateral chest area, and glide and stretch the hand across chest area 2/3/4/5.

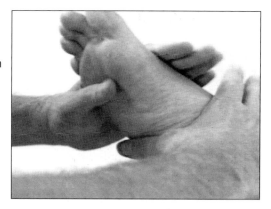

122. Rotations (emotional release)

Make a loose fist with either hand and place the fist on the lung area. Place the palm of the other hand on top of the foot. Rotate both hands slowly with pressure.

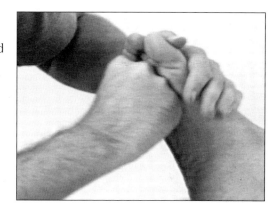

Repeat closing movements 119–122 on the left foot.

Bring both feet together

Put a thumb on the solar plexus point of each foot. Ask the client to take two deep, relaxing breaths in and out. On the third in-breath, press, rotate a little and hold on each solar plexus point. On the out-breath, release the pressure on the solar plexus and pull the top of feet slightly towards you. Repeat another three to five times. (Suggest that the client breathes in everything good and breathes out everything negative). Ask the client to bring breathing back to normal level, to avoid light-headedness.

Stroke the feet away from you and say 'Thank You'.

CHAPTER 2

FOOT REFLEX SEQUENCE (ABRIDGED GUIDE)

Once you have mastered the location of the reflex points, the following will help jog your memory of the sequence order (should you choose to use it). Keep it to hand when performing your first treatments, until you are fully confident.

THE SEQUENCE

THE OPENING MOVEMENTS

Right foot

1.   Rotate the foot

2.   Stretch the achilles

3.   Open and stretch the chest

4.   Solar plexus

Repeat opening movements 1–4 on the left foot (reversing hand positions).

THE RIGHT FOOT

5.   Cervical vertebrae

6.   Head and neck

7.   Brain

8.   Front of neck

9.   Back of neck

10.   Occipital

11.   Ear

12.   Hypothalamus

13.   Pineal

14.   Pituitary

15.   Sinuses

16.   General eye and ear

17. Eye

18. Ear

19. Eustachian tube

20. Balance

21. Shoulder

22. Diaphragm

23. Thyroid

24. Parathyroid

25. Thymus

26. Lungs

27. Gall bladder

28. Liver

29. Stomach/pancreas

30. Duodenum and small intestine

31. Ileo-caecal valve (ICV) and ascending/transverse colon

32. Small intestine/colon helper area

33. Lower back/colon helper area

34. Uterus (female)/prostate (male)

35. Ovary (female)/testes (male)

36. Fallopian tubes (female)/vas deferens (male)

37. Lymphatics

38. Sciatic nerve

39. Shoulder, upper arm, elbow, lower arm, wrist

40. Knee, hip, lower back

41. Chronic back helper area/lower back/sacro-iliac joint and pelvis

42. Bladder

43. Ureter and kidney

44. Adrenals

45. Cervical spine

46. Thoracic spine – downwards

47. Lumbar spine – downwards

48. Coccyx/lower back and sciatic helper area

49. Lumbar spine – upwards

50. Thoracic spine – upwards

51. Thoracic spine – downwards

52. Lumbar spine – downwards

53. Coccyx and sacral area

54. Lumbar spine – upwards

55. Thoracic spine – upwards

56. Spinal nerves – across

57. Lymphatic

58. Chest/breast area

59. Open and stretch chest area

60. Energise zones

61. Rotate, stretch and drain

THE LEFT FOOT

62. Cervical vertebrae

63. Head and neck

64. Brain

65. Front of neck

66. Back of neck

67. Occipital

68. Ear

69. Hypothalamus

70. Pineal

71. Pituitary

72. Sinuses

73. General eye and ear

74. Eye

75. Ear

76. Eustachian tube

77. Balance

78. Shoulder

79. Diaphragm

80. Thyroid

81. Parathyroid

82. Thymus

83. Lungs

84. Cardiac area

85. Heart

86. Spleen

87. Stomach/pancreas

88. Transverse, descending and sigmoid colon

89. Small intestine/colon helper area

90. Lower back/colon helper area

91. Uterus (female)/prostate (male)

92. Ovary (female)/testes (male)

93. Fallopian tubes (female)/vas deferens (male)

94. Lymphatics

95. Sciatic nerve

96. Shoulder, Upper arm, Elbow, Lower arm, Wrist.

97. Knee, hip, lower back

98. Chronic back helper area/lower back/sacro-iliac joint and pelvis

99. Bladder

100. Ureter and kidney

101. Adrenals

102. Cervical spine

103. Thoracic spine – downwards

104. Lumbar spine – downwards

105. Coccyx/lower back and sciatic helper area

106. Lumbar spine – upwards

107. Thoracic spine – upwards

108. Thoracic spine – downwards

109. Lumbar spine – downwards

110. Coccyx and sacral area

111. Lumbar spine – upwards

112. Thoracic spine – upwards

113. Spinal nerves – across

114. Lymphatic

115. Chest/breast area

116. Open and stretch chest area

117. Energise zones

118. Rotate, stretch and drain

THE CLOSING MOVEMENTS

Right Foot

119. Foot massage

120. Spinal release

121. Chest release

122. Rotations (emotional release)

Repeat closing movements 119–122 on the left foot.

Bring both feet together for solar plexus breathing.

CHAPTER 3

Hand reflex sequence (illustrated guide)

Once the foot techniques have been learnt the same techniques can be applied to the hands. When first practising it helps to picture the hand as a short, wide foot with very long toes! (See Figure 2.)

Simplicity in approaching the treatment will help each practitioner develop a unique approach to treating the hands. As the hands are smaller in area to work than the feet, the hand positions for reaching the reflex points can be varied to suit the practitioner, so that the most comfortable position is achieved for both client and practitioner. For example, many more of the points can be worked with the fingers rather than the thumb and many of the reflex areas are smaller so fewer rows are worked (liver is two small rows on the hand rather than three on the foot). A complete hand treatment will also be shorter than a foot treatment, lasting approximately 30 minutes. The hand reflex points, including when to use them, are discussed in detail in Chapter 10.

The zones on the hands follow the same pattern as the feet (see Chapter 6).

The following is a suggested sequence only. It is based on the reflexology chart shown in Figure 2. It is not the only possible sequence, or the only reflexology chart. If you prefer to use a different sequence and chart, then the following guide can still be useful as a reference point for commonly worked reflex areas.

TECHNIQUES USED ARE THE SAME AS FOR THE FOOT:

- **Bites** – crawling movement with pressure of the thumb or fingers. Each movement is known as a 'bite'.

- **Rotate** – clockwise and anticlockwise movements with pressure, applied several times.

- **Press** – a steady, even pressure on a particular area.

Please note that every hand is a different size and shape and therefore any measurements given for reflex locations are approximate. Refer to the illustrations for precise locations.

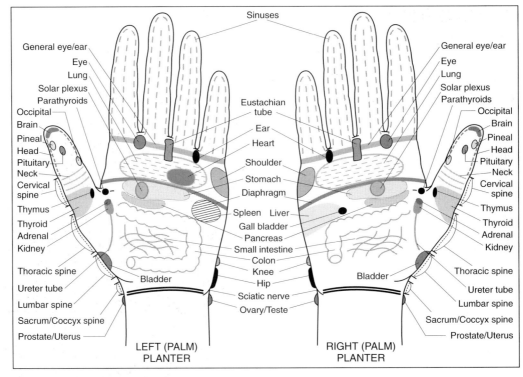

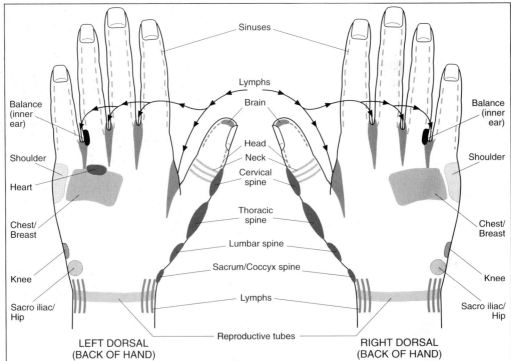

Figure 2. Hand reflex chart

THE SEQUENCE

THE OPENING MOVEMENTS

The reflex points are shown in a suggested order. Do not worry if you prefer a different order. The guide will still be useful for the location of the major reflex points

1. **Rotations**

   Rotate the hand clockwise and anticlockwise.

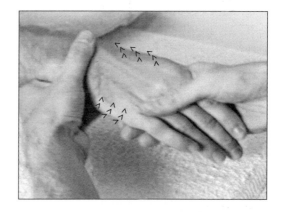

2. **Hand stretch**

   Support the wrist and stretch the hand lightly.

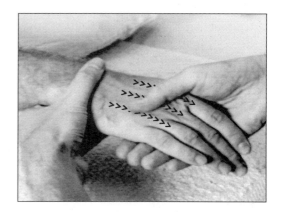

3. **Upper chest stretch**

   Open and stretch the hand with the thumbs across knuckles lightly.

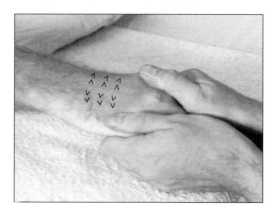

4. Solar plexus

Press and rotate.

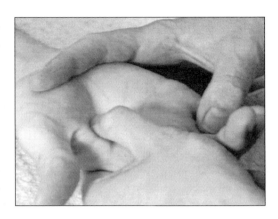

Repeat opening movements 1–4 on the left hand *then return to the right hand.*

THE RIGHT HAND

5. Cervical vertebrae/head and neck/brain

Work with bites up and over the thumb, lateral and medial.

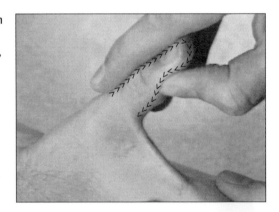

Work the front of the base of the thumb, with bites medial to lateral for the front of the neck and throat.

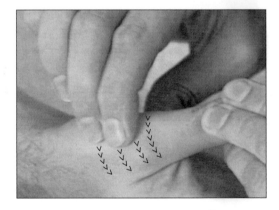

Work the back of the base of the thumb, with bites medial to lateral for the back of the neck.

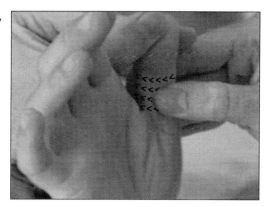

6. Pituitary/pineal/hypothalamus

Press and rotate the pituitary point – the middle of the thumb.

Lift to the medial side of the thumb for pineal and hypothalamus. Press and rotate.

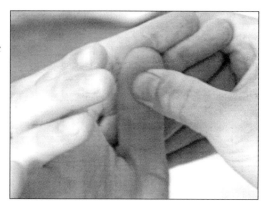

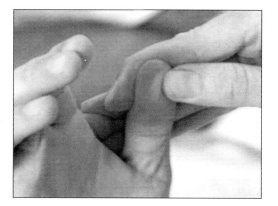

7. Sinuses

Work up in bites each side of all the fingers, then take bites up the centre of each finger (palm side).

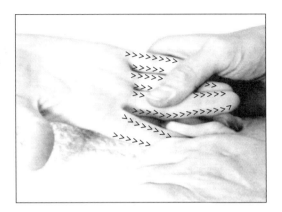

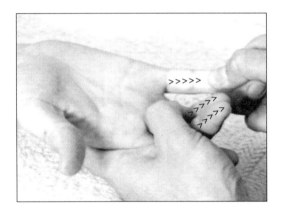

8. Eye/Eustachian/balance/ear

Work in bites across the pads below the base of the fingers, stopping to press and rotate, with the thumb on the palm side and the index finger on top, between 2/3 for eye, 3/4 for Eustachian and between 4/5 for balance and ear.

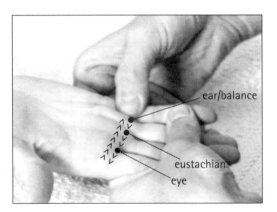

ear/balance

eustachian

eye

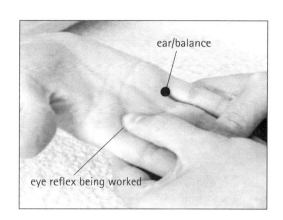

ear/balance

eye reflex being worked

9. **Shoulder**

Work down with bites between 4/5 with pressure on both sides of the hand for about 2.5 cm, then work the palm with pressure and rotations for extra work.

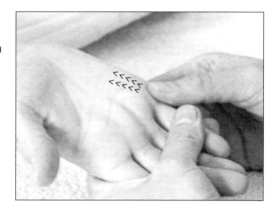

10. **Diaphragm**

Work across the palm and back again with bites.

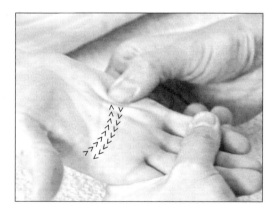

11. Thyroid/parathyroid/thymus

Fill in the thyroid area with bites working with the thumb or index finger, hooking and stimulating on fleshy areas below the thumb.

Press and rotate the parathyroid between 1/2.

Take the bites down for about 2.5 cm for thymus, then hook and press.

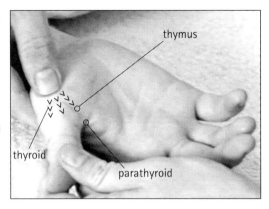

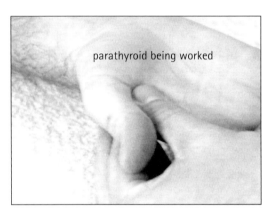

parathyroid being worked

12. Lungs

Work up from the diaphragm with bites between zones 2/3, 3/4 and 4/5.

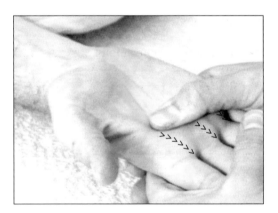

13. Gall bladder/liver

Trace down between 3/4 until just below the diaphragm. Press and rotate for the gall bladder.

Work from the gall bladder to the liver in bites for two rows.

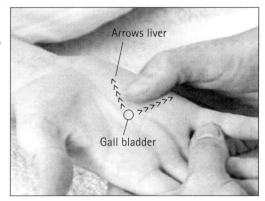

14. Stomach/pancreas

From just below the diaphragm work in bites for two rows across from zone 1 to 3.

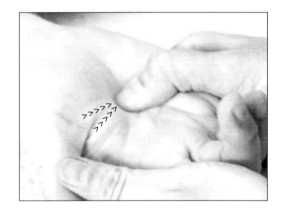

15. Colon/small intestine

Work up with bites between 4/5 for the ascending colon and turn to work with bites across to zone 1 for the transverse colon.

Fill in the small intestine area with bites from zone 4/5 across to zone 1 for two rows, each row lower than the previous.

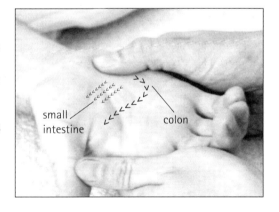

16. Reproductive area

Work the reproductive points on each side of the wrist with pressure.

Work over the wrist with bites for the reproductive tubes.

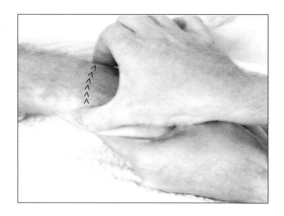

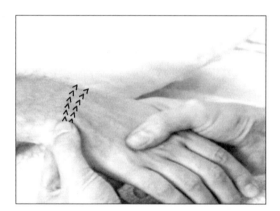

17. Lymphatics

Work around the wrist with bites in two rows.

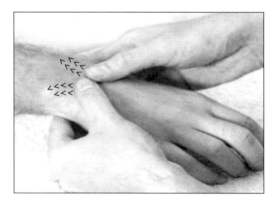

18. Sciatic point

Work the sciatic point with rotations and pressure on zone 1 and zone 5. Then work across with bites to join the two.

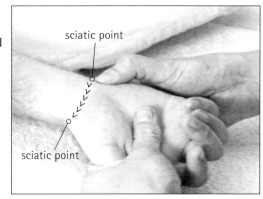

19. Knee, hip, lower back

Work with bites down the side of zone 5 from the base of the finger to the wrist.

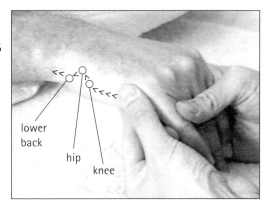

20. Bladder/ureter/kidney/adrenal

Work the bladder with two bites, from the base of zone 1/2.

Then work up the ureter in bites until you reach the kidney and adrenal (level with the base of the thumb). Then press and rotate.

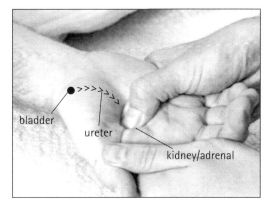

21. Spine (7 cervicals, 12 thoracic, 5 lumbar)

Work the spinal reflexes with bites on the side of zone 1 from the thumb to the base of the palm, then work back again.

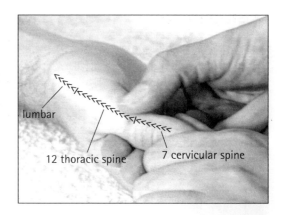

lumbar

12 thoracic spine

7 cervicular spine

22. Lymphatic drainage

Work down between each zone from the base of the fingers for about 3.5 cm, with bites and keeping contact, glide back between the zone to the starting position (between the fingers).

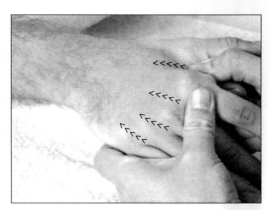

23. Breast/chest

Using the index and second finger, take bites across the zones on top of the hands, from the base of the finger at zone 3 to the base of the finger at zone 5. Work two rows, the second lower than the first.

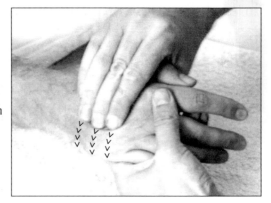

24. Energise zones

Take bites across all the zones (1 to 5) on top of the hands, starting at the wrist and working towards the fingers.

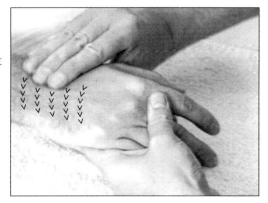

Support and rotate the thumb and fingers.

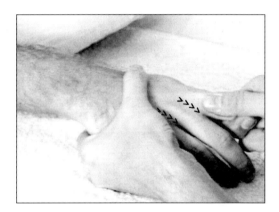

Work down in bites between each finger and thumb about 1.25 cm. Pull back towards the fingers, keeping pressure with the thumb and index finger.

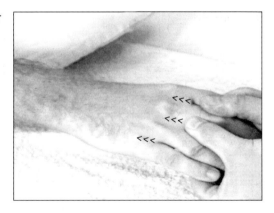

THE LEFT HAND

The left hand follows the same treatment sequence as the right hand up to and including the lungs (sequence numbers 5–12). You may, however, wish to change your hand positions to enable access to the points on this hand. After the lungs the following sequence should be followed:

25. Cardiac area

Work two rows across in bites from zone 5 to 2 – from below the base of the fingers to above the diaphragm line, with the second row lower than the first.

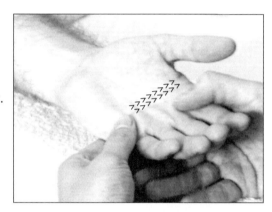

26. Heart reflex

Trace down about 2.5 cm on zone 4 then hook and press. Then press the same area on top of the hand to link together.

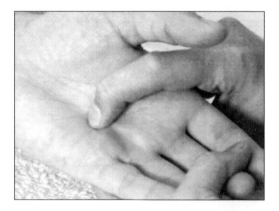

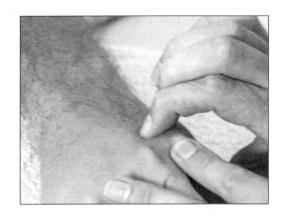

27. Spleen

Locate the point between zones 4/5 (below the diaphragm) then hook in and rotate.

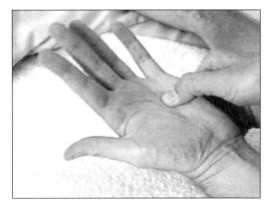

28. Stomach/pancreas

From the spleen work in bites for two rows across to zone 1, with the second row lower than the first.

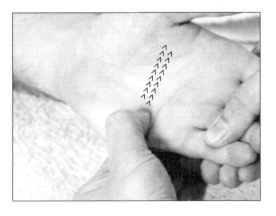

29. Colon/small intestine

From just below the stomach/pancreas point work in bites from zone 1 back to between zones 4/5 for the transverse colon. Hook in and rotate for splenic flexure.

Work down in bites for the descending colon, rotate and press on the sigmoid flexure.

Work across from the sigmoid colon in zone 4/5 to the anus in zone 1.

Fill in the small intestine area with bites from zone 4/5 across to zone 1 for two rows, each row lower than the previous.

After this the left hand again follows the same treatment sequence as the right hand for the reproductives up to and including energising the zones (sequence numbers 16-24).

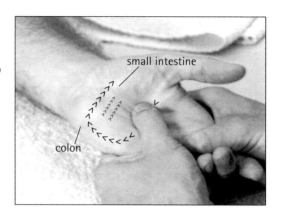

small intestine

colon

SOLAR PLEXUS CLOSING MOVEMENTS

On both hands:

30. Solar plexus breathing

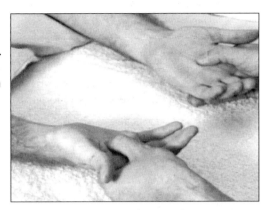

Place a thumb on each solar plexus point. Ask the client to take two deep relaxing breaths in and out. On the third in-breath press, rotate a little and hold on each solar plexus point. On the out-breath, release pressure on the solar plexus.

Repeat another three to five times. (Suggest that the client breathes in everything good and breathes out everything negative). Ask the client to bring breathing back to normal level, to avoid light-headedness.

Stroke the hands away from you and say 'Thank You'.

A hand treatment can be very relaxing, especially as the hands are not usually rested or manipulated. It is therefore essential that the client rests the hands for 10 minutes after the treatment and does not drive or operate machinery during this time.

The treatment is also beneficial to those who use their hands a lot in a profession such as keyboarders, musicians, masseurs, osteopaths, podiatrists, reflexologists, painters, carpenters etc, as it can help to combat the effects of repetitive use and keep the hands fit and healthy.

CHAPTER 4

What is Reflexology?

Of course *you* will know what reflexology is because you are interested in it, are studying it or perhaps having treatments! There are many descriptions of reflexology, all of which vary in length, detail and philosophy but a good short description is:

> *'reflexology is pressure massage to the feet or hands in order to stimulate the reflex points and bring about a balance of the eight bodily systems in order for the body to work together in harmony and unison and thus creating a feeling of well-being and optimum health.'*

This description covers the main points and is short enough to remember. It also means that you sound professional when describing reflexology to other people. Professionalism, even as a student, is very important in promoting not only reflexology in general but your own practice in particular. As you begin to mention your study of reflexology to others they will be interested to know what it involves. By having a short, confident description at the ready you will come across as knowledgeable and professional – after all, the people who are interested in your training today may be your clients of tomorrow.

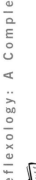

Task 1 • Give a brief description of reflexology.

Task 2 • Why is it important to be clear about what reflexology is.

The eight bodily systems, which reflexology helps to balance are:

Bodily system	Example reflex area falling within the system:
Skeletal	Spine
Muscular	Muscles in the neck
Neurological	Brain
Respiratory	Lungs
Digestive	Stomach
Endocrine	Adrenal gland
Genito urinary	Bladder
Vascular	Heart

The human body is completely reflected in the feet in a three-dimensional form, and a point on the foot which relates to an area of the body is called a *reflex*.

By applying pressure with the hands to the reflex areas of the feet the reflexologist can locate blockages and imbalances of the reflexes and zone pathways which, through treatment, can be corrected, thus restoring the flow of the body's natural healing energies and aiding a return to optimum health.

 Task 3 • **Give an example of a body structure or organ that falls within each bodily system.**

Reflexology is a safe, natural, non-invasive therapy. No medication or implements of any kind are used.

HOW DOES IT WORK?

Reflexology is a form of complementary therapy. This means it can be used by itself or together with other forms of complementary or orthodox/allopathic treatment. It is not an alternative to medical treatment nor is it a way of diagnosing ailments or providing specific cures. It is a therapy that helps to release a client's own healing potential.

There are many theories why reflexology works as a form of complementary treatment. Some possibilities are:

1. Stimulation of some of the 2,000 neurotransmitters between the nerve endings of the feet and the body.

2. Influence of the meridians (acupressure points, chi energy etc.).

3. Polarity (electrically charged energy flows).

4. Zones – influence of the body through the zone mapping system (see later chapters).

5. Energy exchange from practitioner to client.

6. TLC (tender loving care). The healing physical touch.

WHAT CAN IT DO?

1. Reflexology increases blood circulation, aiding the carriage of essential hormones, oxygen and nutrients necessary for cell life.

2. It improves lymphatic circulation to aid the dispersal of waste products and stimulates the immune system.

3. It aids the relief of congestion and other deposits in the feet (uric acids, calcium deposits) leading to increased circulation.

4. It offers a chance to rest – the act of slowing down and actually taking time out for the treatment.

WHAT ARE THE BENEFITS?

- Relaxation

- Pain relief

- Improved circulation

- Improved muscle tone

- Stimulation of immune system

- Improved elimination (detoxifying)

- Manipulation of the foot itself (joints, muscles, ligaments etc.)

- Encourages body to heal

- Psychological comfort

- Nerve stimulation

- Balance of mind, body and spirit

- Human touch and interaction

There is no one simplistic explanation as to why reflexology works. It can be seen to work on several levels of the individual – physical, mental, spiritual and emotional.

We have seen on the previous pages that we are working on many levels, and it is therefore not uncommon for a client to experience some reactions to the treatment. In later chapters we will discuss the reasons for such reactions in more detail. Below is a list of some of the most common reactions during or after a treatment:

- Feeling hot

- Feeling cold

- Sweaty palms

- Increased urination

- Increased energy

- Decreased energy (feeling tired)

 Task 4 • List four actual reactions that a client may have during or after receiving a reflexology treatment.

CHAPTER 5

The history of reflexology

There are many theories regarding the development of reflexology. It could have developed in many different parts of the world at different times. Its later development could have been due to many people and factors. However, it is generally accepted that certain main events have led to reflexology as we know it today. Below is a list of the important events in date order:

2330 BC   Wall carving on Egyptian Tomb of the physician to the king. Depicted pressure massage to the feet and hands.

332 BC   Egyptian Scrolls spread knowledge to Greece, Arabia and the Roman Empire. Monks from India bring knowledge of massage and footwork to China.

AD 1017   Dr Wang Wei (China) cast a bronze figure marking important acupuncture points on the body. Pressure on the feet used in conjunction with acupuncture needles and meridian lines.

1582   Dr Adamus and Dr A'tatis, eminent European physicians, wrote about zone therapy in a book published in this year.

1893   Sir Henry Head (UK) proved the neurological (nerve) relationship between pressure applied to the skin and internal organs.

1906   Sir Charles Sherrington (UK) showed that the brain, spinal cord and reflex pathways control the activities of the body. He showed that nerves could transmit signals around the body. He established that nerves coordinate body functions. He published a book, *The Integrative Action of the Nervous System*. His achievements were recognised by his peers when he was awarded the Nobel prize for science.

1913–20   Dr William Fitzgerald, an American ear, nose and throat surgeon, developed a technique later to be described by medical journalist Dr Edwin Bowers as 'zone therapy' (1917). European sources and new research on the nervous system probably influenced him. It is also possible that the native American Indian foot and bodywork tradition influenced his views. Fitzgerald experimented with pain thresholds and pressure points. He discovered that pressure applied to the body could have an anaesthetic effect on other parts removed from the pressure site. He documented the division of the body into ten longitudinal sections. The interrelationship between certain points of the body and organs removed from the point was explored.

1920–30   Further development by American doctors George Starr White and Joe Riley. Riley with his wife Elizabeth developed 'Hook Work'. He developed the first diagrams of foot reflex points and reflex points of the ear. The use of the reflex points of the ear is known as *Auriculotherapy*. He developed eight horizontal zones. The Rileys ran a therapy school teaching zone therapy and published a book, *Zone Therapy Simplified*.

1930–38   Eunice Ingham, an American therapy assistant to Dr Riley, further developed the zone therapy system by charting the relationship of the zones to the feet and evolving the 'map' of the body through the feet.

1938   Eunice Ingham wrote *Stories the Feet Can Tell* and became known as a foot therapist. She further developed and refined the technique now known as *reflexology*, sharing her findings and experiences with her colleagues and students.

1963   Eunice Ingham wrote *Stories the Feet Have Told*.

1966   Doreen Bayly (UK), a former student of Eunice Ingham, pioneered Reflexology in England.

1966–74   German reflexologist Hanne Marquardt, a student of Eunice Ingham, developed transverse zones. First practitioner to work in Germany with pressure on the feet only. Trained the medically qualified in reflexology. She published a book, *Zone Therapy of the Feet*.

1984   Doreen Bayly (UK) published *Reflexology Today*.

The Association of Reflexologists (UK) founded as an independent reflexology organisation.

1985   Reflexology accepted as a form of complementary medicine by the ICM (Institute for Complementary Medicine) in the UK.

Task 5 • Briefly describe the major contributions made to reflexology by the following people:
    a) Dr William Fitzgerald
    b) Dr Joe Shelby Riley
    c) Hanne Marquardt.

Task 6 • a) Describe the important principal established by Sir Charles Sherrington (1861–1952) in his work, The *Integrative Action of the Nervous System*, which later went on to win him the Nobel prize.
    b) Who is widely regarded as having introduced reflexology into the United Kingdom?
    c) Approximately when did this take place?

MODERN–DAY DEVELOPMENT

Reflexology has enjoyed an enormous increase in public interest in recent years. This is good news for practitioners as it keeps the therapy in the public eye and generates new clients. There are several factors that have increased interest in reflexology:

- Increasing interest in the media and the public at large

- Growing attention from the medical profession

- Increased pressure to validate the therapy

- A growing body of research into the therapy and the growth of properly conducted research trials

- Efforts by the Government to bring about some sort of regulation of complementary therapies

- The development of National Occupational Standards for the therapy

- The growth of standard training aims and examinations.

- A debate within the European Community about the 'harmonisation' of complementary therapies.

- Availability of detailed information via the Internet.

Reflexology has also derived other therapies. These therapies are based upon reflexology but offer completely different treatments. Two examples are metamorphic technique and vacuflex.

METAMORPHIC TECHNIQUE

A very light touch treatment which concentrates on the spine and head reflexes on the feet, head and hands. The metamorphic philosophy relates these areas to foetal development.

VACUFLEX

A mechanical treatment where vacuum boots are placed on the feet. When removed, the feet are examined for areas of redness. These areas are then further treated with a massage machine or by hand.

Task 7 • a) Give two experiences/sources of knowledge that may have influenced Dr William Fitzgerald in his development of zone therapy.
b) Name three influences that are affecting the development of our therapy today.

CULTURAL DIFFERENCES – EASTERN REFLEXOLOGY

Modern reflexology techniques differ across the world but most share the general principal of pressure massage with the hands to the reflex areas of the feet. The exception to this is the Eastern method of reflexology also known as the Chinese or Rwo Shur method. This method involves the use of short sticks or the knuckles to apply pressure. The pressure is also very hard!

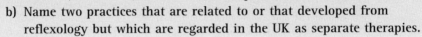

Task 8 •   a) Give two ways in which the Eastern method of reflexology (e.g. Chinese, Rwo Shur) differs from that practised in the West.
   b) Name two practices that are related to or that developed from reflexology but which are regarded in the UK as separate therapies.

CHAPTER 6

Chart theory, zones and cross reflexes

AN IMPORTANT NOTE ABOUT REFLEXOLOGY CHARTS

The most confusing aspect of learning the reflexology sequence is the variety of charts and diagrams available, many of which seem to vary in their depiction of the location of some reflex points. There will also be a variety of suggestions as to the order of the treatment.

The important thing to remember about reflexology charts, treatment sequences, zones and cross reflexes is that they represent a map. The reason for looking at any map is to get to the right location in the most efficient manner. If you travel the same route enough times you will no longer need the map, indeed you may even find different routes to the same location. You may then decide to create your own map to share the new routes. It is also possible that other people reading the same map will look at it differently and decide on a different location by another route. So it is with reflexology charts. It is best to stick with your preferred chart in order to learn the sequence and the location of reflex areas, but always be open to different approaches and techniques.

There are also some other explanations as to the variation in reflex charts:

1. The foot is not a perfect reflection of the shape of the body and therefore the location of certain reflex points is dependent on the anatomical interpretation of the foot.

2. Personal experience of performing reflexology may draw practitioners to vary their technique and create differing charts.

3. In rare circumstances there can be quite wide variations in the placement of some organs in the body of different individuals.

4. There may be more than one reflex area for some parts of the body, or reflex areas on the foot overlap and overlay each other, just as structures in the body do.

5. Copyright restrictions.

CHARTS – HOW TO USE THEM

This book provides a reflex chart in Chapter 1 (see figure 1) for guidance only. You may of course use your preferred chart for the reasons discussed above. Chapter 1 also gives an example reflex sequence and illustrations of commonly taught reflex points.

There is some common terminology used when referring to reflex locations on the foot:

- Dorsal   The top of the foot (i.e. the part of the foot you can see when looking down).

- Plantar   The bottom (sole) of the foot (i.e. the part of the foot that you stand on).

- Medial   Imagine the body has a line directly down its centre. This is known as the medial line. Therefore if a reflex is 'towards the medial' it means towards the middle of the body. For example, the medial side of the big toe would be the side that faces in towards the centre of the body.

- Lateral   Is the opposite of the above. A reflex 'towards the lateral' means towards the outside of the body or away from the medial line. For example, the lateral side of the big toe would be the side that is next to the second toe because this is nearest the outside of the body.

The purpose of all reflexology charts is to show the location of the *reflex points*. These are the areas of the body that are reflected on the foot. A reflexology chart will generally show the reflex areas by highlighting the shape of the reflex point or area and showing different colours for each reflex point or each point within the same bodily system (remember the eight bodily systems in Chapter 4). The best way to learn while training is to stick with your preferred chart.

Some of the reflex areas shown on charts and diagrams closely resemble the actual shape of the body. For example, the spine and the medial arch of the foot, and the bladder reflex and the bladder.

Task 9 • a) **On a template of the right foot, using your preferred reflex chart, draw in the location of the following six reflexes and label each one:**
Adrenals   Bladder   Hip
Pituitary   Shoulder   Sinuses
    b) **Name two reflexes that may be accessed on the dorsal surface of the foot as well as the more normal position on the plantar surface.**

ZONES – WHAT THEY MEAN AND HOW WE USE THEM

As mentioned in Chapter 5 Dr William Fitzgerald (1872–1942) was the founder of zone therapy. In his book *Zone Therapy* he remarked:

'A form of treatment by means of pressure point massage was known in India and China some 5000 years ago. This knowledge appears however to have been lost or forgotten, perhaps it was set aside in favour of acupuncture, which emerged as the stronger growth from the same route'.

Zone therapy is an important concept for reflexologists because it gives us the 'zones' that divide the feet. The theory divides the body into ten longitudinal zones (see figure 3):

- Zone 1 runs from the top of the head through the centre of the forehead and nose and onwards through the centre of the body, branching off to the thumbs and big toes.

- Zone 2 runs from the top of the head, down through the eye and onwards through the body to the first finger and second toe.

- Zone 3 runs from the top of the head, through the eye and down to the second finger and third toe.

- Zone 4 runs down from the top of the head, through the middle ear and down to the third finger and fourth toe.

- Zone 5 runs from the top of the head, takes in the external ear and continues down to the little or fourth finger and fifth toe.

The five zones lie on either side of the body with zone one coming together in the centre of the body to form a middle or median line.

The zones are like segments of the body and are not to be confused with acupuncture meridian pathways. (See Figure 3).

All the body zones end in the feet. Imagine drawing a straight line between each toe down to the heel. These are the body zones reflected on the feet (see figure 4). The big toe represents the head area. This is where all five zones combine. All organs, glands and nervous systems fall into these zones, hence a complete map of the body can be shown on the feet. By pressing certain areas within a zone on the feet it is possible to affect other parts of the body. Reflexologists believe that energy travels through the zones, connecting every part of the body that lie in the same zone.

The zone references are three dimensional; each section includes the inside of the body from front to back. Therefore the reflex points are to be found in the front as well as in the back and on both the upper and lower part. (See Figure 4).

Task 10 • a) Give two explanations for the fact that there are many different charts, with reflexes in different locations.
b) Briefly describe zone theory.
c) How is the arrangement of zones on the big toes different from the rest of the foot?
d) Why do reflexologists often work the kidneys to help an eye disorder?

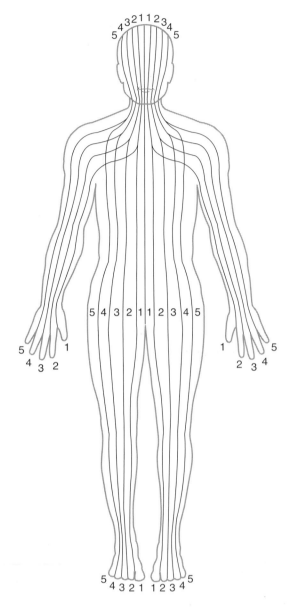

Figure 3. The longitudinal zones of the body

TRANSVERSE ZONES

In addition to longitudinal division the body and, therefore, the foot, is horizontally partitioned to enable location of the body parts. The horizontal divisions of both the feet and body are known as *transverse* or *lateral zones*. The three main lines used on the foot are:

1. The shoulder line

2. The diaphragm line

3. The hip/pelvic line

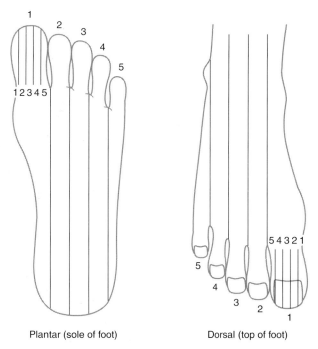

Plantar (sole of foot) Dorsal (top of foot)

Figure 4. The longitudinal zones of the feet

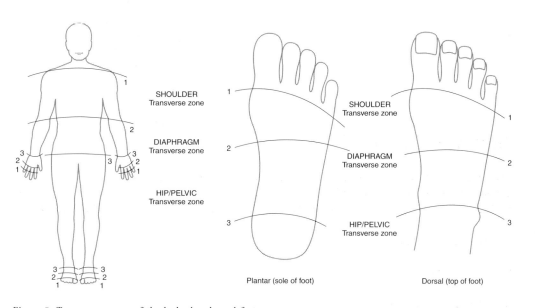

SHOULDER
Transverse zone

DIAPHRAGM
Transverse zone

HIP/PELVIC
Transverse zone

SHOULDER
Transverse zone

DIAPHRAGM
Transverse zone

HIP/PELVIC
Transverse zone

Plantar (sole of foot) Dorsal (top of foot)

Figure 5. Transverse zones of the body, hands and feet

Task 11 • a) Name three reflexes that occur between the diaphragm line and the shoulder line.
   b) Name the longitudinal zone(s) in which each of the following reflexes lie: eye, lung, pancreas, adrenal.

CROSS REFLEXES AND REFERRAL AREAS

As zones extend throughout the whole body, the arms and legs are made up of the same zones. A relationship will, therefore, exist between the right arm and right leg, and the left arm and left leg and the joints in these limbs. These 'parallel' or 'zone-related' areas are more commonly known as cross reflexes (see figure 6). Examples of cross reflexes are:

- Hand to foot
- Hip to shoulder

- Knee to elbow
- Ankle to wrist

Cross reflexes can be used to affect bodily areas where, for various reasons, a direct treatment on the foot cannot be applied, such as:

- injury or infection to foot reflexes

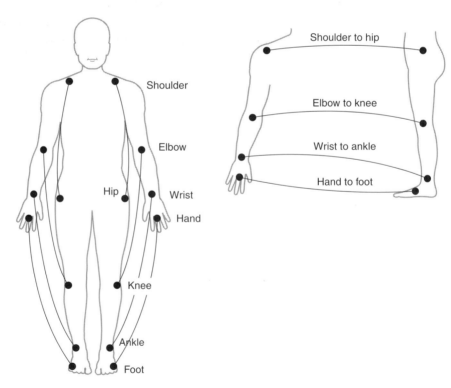

Figure 6. Cross reflex areas of the body

- to reinforce work on the foot

- for client homework between treatments

- unable to access the foot for practical reasons (i.e. on an aircraft).

Treatment of these areas is known as 'referral'. For example, the referral zone of the elbow would be the knee, etc.

Connections between parallel zones can be complex. The horizontal and transverse sectors can interact and weave many inter-crossing areas. Looking at the body through the zones rather than parts and organs enables a complete picture of the whole person to be formed.

Task 12 • a) What is a cross reflex (also known as a referral area)?
  b) Give four examples of cross reflexes.
  c) Give two reasons why you might use a cross reflex.

Task 13 • a) On a right foot template draw in and label the lateral/transverse zones of the feet on both plantar and dorsal aspects.
  b) On a left foot template draw in and label the longitudinal zones.
  c) On a left foot template, using your preferred reflex chart, draw in the location of the following reflexes and label each one:

| Stomach | Cervical vertebrae | Spleen | Heart/cardiac area |
| Kidney | Upper lymphatics | Sigmoid colon | Prostate |

CHAPTER 7

Practical reflexology – the five-step approach

PRACTICAL REFLEXOLOGY SKILLS

Now we know what reflexology is and where it comes from, it is time to concentrate on the practical skills needed to give a good treatment. Remember that your skills will improve only with practice and that you should take the time to use the techniques you have learnt on as many pairs of feet as you can. Don't worry if you are not perfect, it is your interaction with the client and the experience of working that will improve your technique.

Refer to Chapter 1 for an example reflex sequence and illustrations of commonly taught reflex areas.

When treating clients think of the five learning steps.

- Step 1 Learn the treatment sequence and reflex points

- Step 2 Learn the basic hand movements needed to access the reflex points

- Step 3 Learn the pressure needed and when to vary it

- Step 4 Learn to interpret the sensations you feel, and what they may mean

- Step 5 Learn to vary the sequence and the pressure for each individual, based on the feedback from the reflexes.

These five steps are crucial for an effective treatment. Think of them as a continuous, circular process.

 STEPS

Here are the five steps in detail:

STEP 1   LEARN THE TREATMENT SEQUENCE

Reflexologists use a *treatment sequence*. A sequence is a way of remembering what part of the foot to treat next. Just as we discussed the variety of charts available in Chapter 6, the

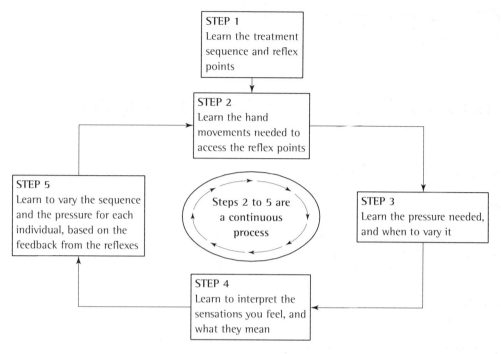

Figure 7 The five learning steps

same applies to sequences. Some sequences will start on the right foot, complete the entire foot and then treat the left foot. Some will move continuously from one foot to the other and others will start on the left foot. Starting on either foot will be equally effective, but there are several reasons for the different approaches:

⇒ Starting on the right foot rebalances the physical side first (left brain), before moving on to the emotional side (right brain). Working the right foot first also follows the natural flow of the colon (large intestine), which begins on the right foot and expels on the left.

⇒ Starting on the left foot opens the more receptive side of the brain; otherwise the body might reject the stimulation

⇒ Starting on the client's dominant side (i.e. depending on whether they are right handed or left handed) rebalances the stronger parts first.

⇒ Working both feet simultaneously balances systems across the body.

Whichever approach is used the client will certainly feel the beneficial effects of a treatment!

Chapter 1 suggests a practical sequence. This does not replace your preferred sequence but it is useful for self-study or for those interested in other sequences. It also gives useful information about reflex points – whatever order you treat them.

STEP 2 LEARN THE BASIC MOVEMENTS

All reflexology sequences need three basic types of movement:

⇒ Rotation, as in the solar plexus.

   Movements in a clockwise and anticlockwise direction, with pressure.

⇒ Bites or walking/crawling/triggering, as in the seven cervical vertebrae and the head and neck area.

   Bending the thumb and moving in 'bites' across the skin, with pressure to trigger points.

⇒ Hooking, as in the thymus.

   Sideways pressure with the thumb.

 Task 14 • Does it make any difference which foot is used to start the treatment? State the reason why you begin on your chosen foot.

STEP 3 LEARN THE PRESSURE NEEDED AND WHEN TO VARY IT

With any of the above movements pressure must be applied. The pressure should be firm enough for the client to feel but not to the point where your hands feel strained with the pressure, or your client is pulling their foot away in discomfort. Glance at your client regularly during the treatment to ensure the pressure is comfortable for them.

It is also important to use lighter pressure than normal in certain circumstances:

⇒ Elderly or infirm clients are more vulnerable to pressure and may have bone degenerative conditions such as osteoporosis.

⇒ Young children are still 'developing' on a physical level as well as emotionally and as such are more vulnerable to reactions to the treatment.

⇒ Clients who have recently undergone major surgery need time to recover and are not ready for the effects of full pressure for at least six weeks.

⇒ On clients who show a painful (rather than a sensitive or uncomfortable) reaction to any reflex point.

⇒ On clients in situations where you are unsure of how they will react to a first treatment, possibly because of information gathered during the initial consultation.

STEP 4 LEARN TO INTERPRET THE SENSATIONS YOU FEEL
AND WHAT THEY MAY MEAN

During the treatment you may feel various sensations over different parts of the foot, for example:

⇒ Crystals or grittiness that feel like grains of sugar or sand

⇒ Changes in muscular tone

⇒ Swollen areas

⇒ 'Empty' or hollow-feeling degenerated areas

⇒ Flexibility or rigidity

⇒ Joint mobility

⇒ Change of temperature

⇒ 'Bubbling' or 'popping' of reflex areas

⇒ Hard areas

⇒ Soft, spongy areas

⇒ Resistive 'solid' areas

⇒ Dry or moist areas

⇒ Lumpiness

⇒ Pulsing sensation

⇒ Sensation of congestion or adhesion of tissue

You will not necessarily feel any or all of the above sensations when treating a client, but if you do they should be viewed only as 'clues' to the client's state of health.

Reflexologists experience the sensations of reflex imbalances in very personal ways and you may feel different responses to those listed above.

Task 15 • a) Describe four situations in which you might lighten your normal pressure.
b) Reflexologists make observations and assessments from the feel of the foot. List six different sensations that may be felt by the therapist through touch during the course of a treatment or several treatments.

MAKING SENSE OF THE SENSATIONS

The sensations that may be felt during a treatment can also be known as 'sensitive' or 'out of balance' areas and can indicate:

⇒ an energy imbalance in the area

⇒ an ongoing physical problem

⇒ a temporary or passing state of tension or stress in the area

⇒ a 'memory' held in the reflex of an old problem, now gone

⇒ a past condition that has been suppressed and now resolved

⇒ an area of weakness or vulnerability in the body that may give rise to future problems

⇒ an emotional or mental state

⇒ the effect of medication on particular areas of the body.

These interpretations should be viewed only in conjunction with the client's presenting problems and case history, which will be discussed in a later chapter. You should not rely on the interpretations of the reflex sensations *alone* when formulating a treatment plan.

 Task 16 • Give five possible reasons why a particular reflex might be sensitive or out of balance.

STEP 5   LEARN TO VARY THE SEQUENCE AND THE PRESSURE FOR EACH INDIVIDUAL, BASED ON THE FEEDBACK OF THE REFLEXES

During a treatment you will be thinking about the following: the treatment sequence and reflex points, the hand movements needed to access the points, the pressure applied to the points, the feel and interpretation of the reflex points and the client's reaction, your assessment of the sensation of certain reflex points and whether it indicates, taking into account the client's case history, that it may be out of balance. The final step of the practical treatment process is to assess the above information and decide which reflex points require extra attention. This extra attention can be given in several ways:

⇒ Taking smaller crawling movements as you cross the area

⇒ Passing over the area from several directions

⇒ Varying the angle of your approach to a point

⇒ Working over the area several times

⇒ Pressing and rotating on the area for a longer time

⇒ Returning to rework the area throughout the treatment

⇒ Using alternative/additional techniques

⇒ Avoiding certain areas or treating areas with lighter pressure

⇒ Returning to the area at the end of treatment to do more detailed work on it

⇒ Showing the client how they can reinforce the work on their hands at home

⇒ Holding with firm pressure for longer. Stimulating trigger points for longer.

 Task 17 • Many practitioners give extra attention to reflex areas felt to be out of balance. Describe three ways in which you might include such work in your treatment session.

CHAPTER 8

Contraindications

WHAT IS A CONTRAINDICATION?

Contraindication means 'against-treatment'. It is a general phrase used to indicate a group of conditions that should not receive a reflexology treatment or that a treatment may be given but caution must be exercised.

Contraindications exist in order to prevent the possibility of the reflexology treatment causing deterioration of the condition itself.

The practitioner's common sense should be used at all times and treatment postponed if there is any doubt as to the presence of a contraindication. A reflexologist should treat only within the level of their competence; in other words if you do not feel confident treating a client with a certain condition do not treat them.

MAJOR CONTRAINDICATIONS

Reflexology is a very safe form of treatment but in order to protect both the practitioner and the client it is advisable not to treat the following major contraindication.

Condition	Reason
Deep vein thrombosis (DVT)	The strong effect on the circulatory systems caused by a reflexology treatment may worsen
Phlebitis	such conditions. It is absolutely forbidden to treat persons with blood clots due to the
Blood Clots	possibility of movement of the blood clot in the direction of the lungs, heart and brain.

Task 18 • a) What do you understand is meant by the term 'contraindication'?
  b) Name two conditions that some practitioners consider to be major contraindications to reflexology treatment.

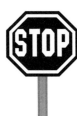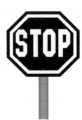

MAJOR CONTRAINDICATION:
THROMBOSIS, PHLEBITIS, BLOOD CLOTS

THROMBOSIS

Formation of a *thrombus* (blood clot) within a blood vessel. Can occur in arteries or deep veins (DVT) (commonly in legs)

CAUSES:

IN ARTERIES	IN DEEP VEINS
Clotting encouraged by build-up of fatty deposits Smoking Diabetes High blood pressure Upset of the body's coagulation mechanisms due to inactivity Slow blood flow to a particular area due to inactivity	Sluggish blood flow Liver disease Age/Obesity/Oral contraceptive Slow blood flow to a particular area due to inactivity

SYMPTOMS

May cause no symptoms until it impairs the blood flow enough to reduce the function of an organ or tissue	May cause no symptoms until it impairs the blood flow enough to reduce the function of an organ or tissue **EXCEPT leg may show swelling, pain, discoloration, tenderness and ulceration**

PHLEBITIS

Inflammation of part of a vein near to the surface of the body, with a clot formation in the affected segment. Also called THROMBOPHLEBITIS.

SYMPTOMS

Swelling and redness along the affected segment. Extreme tenderness. Can lead to deep vein thrombosis

From the above it can be seen that thrombosis can be more difficult to detect than phlebitis – detectable signs are shown in **bold**. *ALWAYS ask* a new client if they suffer from thrombosis or phlebitis

Figure 8 Major contraindications

Reflexology: A Complete Guide

OTHER CONDITIONS OR SITUATIONS

It is also generally agreed that clients with the following conditions can be treated but with a degree of caution:

Condition	Reason
Serious medical condition	Any serious medical condition currently being treated by a medically qualified person without first obtaining that person's consent
Immediately prior to or directly after major surgery	Treatment should not be given immediately prior to or directly after major surgery as to do so may change or cover up symptoms and mask important information. If an operation is postponed for several months (e.g kidney stones, stomach ulcers, orthopaedic procedures) it is acceptable to establish a treatment process. Treatment immediately before or after minor surgery (e.g. local anaesthetic procedures) is acceptable with medical consent
Pregnancy	Reflexology itself is not a danger to a stable pregnancy but should not be undertaken where any element of risk is involved, for example a history of unstable pregnancies or miscarriages
Infectious or contagious conditions	In severe infectious conditions the increase of circulation caused by a reflexology treatment may spread the infection. Treatment can be undertaken *following* the acute state of the infectious disease in order to strengthen those areas which have been affected
Abnormal temperature	Again, the increase of circulation may worsen the condition

Condition	Reason
Directly over an area of varicose vein or varicose eczema	Pressure on the vein is likely to worsen the condition. Light pressure may be applied to the surrounding area
Massive drug intake	Massive potent medication, which is taken daily and affects the systems of the body, may counteract with the reflexology treatment. Caution must be used and if in doubt the permission of the client's GP obtained
Recreational drugs and alchohol	Do not treat if client is obviously under the effects of drugs or alchohol at the time of the treatment. Otherwise a treatment can be offered but be aware that long-term drugs use could affect the sensitivity of the reflexes
Unstable blood pressure	This applies to those persons who suffer from EXTREME FLUCTUATIONS and sharp changes in blood pressure rather than high or low
Heart attacks	Persons who have suffered a heart attack should not be treated for some time in order for the heart muscle to recover. Treatment should not begin until at least three months after the attack. Earlier treatments may be undertaken with the consent of the consultant
Severe local infections of the feet, injuries or degenerative bone conditions	Direct contact with injured tissue will often aggravate and exacerbate the condition. Osteoporosis in an advanced form should not be treated by reflexology. A foot with a serious infection or with infected sores (including gangrene), recent breaks or trauma should not be treated.

Condition	Reason
Cancer	Several types of cancer should not be treated by the reflexologist as the level of malignancy and the risk of worsening the condition is high, for example lymphoma (cancer of the lymphatic system). Other conditions where the person is clearly terminally ill and in severe pain may benefit from the reflexology treatment bringing some alleviation of pain and the side effects of drug treatment. It may also make the remaining time easier to bear. It is always advisable to check with a cancer patient's GP before undertaking a reflexology treatment
After a heavy meal	Energy is concentrated in the stomach following a meal and the patient may feel nausea or experience stomach aches or discomfort if treated too soon afterwards. Allow about two hours after consumption before undertaking treatment
Children, the frail and the elderly	Work with lighter pressure over the reflexes of children and young people approaching puberty. Care must also be taken on the degree of pressure applied to the feet of people who are elderly or frail.
Negative reactions	If contact with the person's feet produces a harsh reaction for no discernible reason and they continue to feel very uncomfortable during the first few minutes of treatment, and a worsening reaction to touch in general is shown, discontinue the treatment immediately. If the same reaction occurs on a following treatment DO NOT treat this patient.

Condition	Reason
HIV and AIDS	Treatment should be applied as normal, remembering these clients may need extra emotional support. Be aware of organisations that can support the client. Do not treat if there are open cuts or sores on the feet. Once these have healed treatment can resume.
Menstruation	Treatment should be applied with lighter pressure than normal (over the reproductive reflexes) during the first few days of a period and avoided completely if menstruation is very heavy.

NEGATIVE REACTIONS

As mentioned in the above table it is possible for some clients to experience a negative or hypersensitive reaction to a reflexology treatment. This may show itself in the client by any or all of the following reactions:

- extreme sweating
- dizziness
- faintness

- nausea
- uncontrollable shaking
- hyperventilation

This sort of reaction is very rare but if it occurs treatment should be stopped immediately. The client should be kept warm and allowed time to recover. If the symptoms persist advise your client to see a GP. These hypersensitive reactions could be an indication of an underlying condition or may be unrelated to any other conditions, merely an indicator that reflexology is not the right treatment for this client. This sort of reaction is very rare.

Task 19 • a) **Name two conditions that may indicate caution is required during treatment; give the condition and reason for caution in each case.**
b) **Give two indications that show a client may be having a hypersensitive response during treatment.**

REMEMBER!

Reflexology is a safe, non-invasive treatment with only one definite contraindication, but several conditions that may require a degree of caution. It is extremely rare, some would say impossible, for the treatment to contribute to or cause any serious condition – but if in doubt avoid the related areas or postpone treatment.

The feet

STRUCTURE OF THE FEET

In reflexology we are concerned with three main elements of the structure of the feet: joints, arches and bones.

JOINTS

There are two types of joint in the feet:

- Hinge joints in the ankle and toes

- Gliding joints between tarsals, or between tarsals and metatarsals.

ARCHES

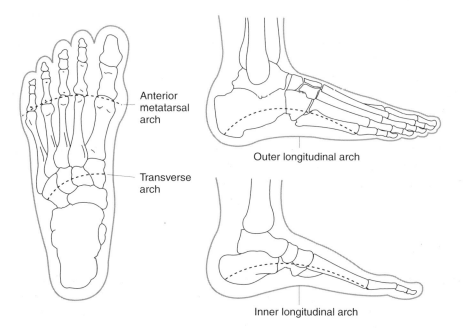

Anterior metatarsal arch

Transverse arch

Outer longitudinal arch

Inner longitudinal arch

Figure 9. The arches of the feet

The arches of the feet (see figure 9):

- bear the weight of the body and distribute it across the foot

- absorb the shock of movement

- lock and become rigid when standing to enable the foot to support the weight of the body

- act as a lever to propel the body forward in motion

- balance the body

- allow flexibility of movement.

BONES

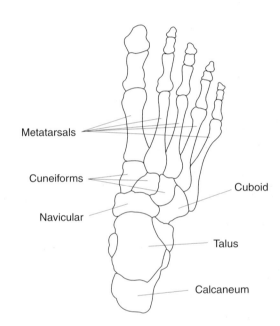

Figure 10. The bones of the feet

The cuneiforms, navicular, cuboid, talus and calcaneum form the *Tarsus* of the foot.

There are 26 bones on each foot. The main weight-bearing bones are the talus (ankle bone), calcaneum (heel bone) and the first metatarsal head. The Achilles tendon is attached to the calcaneum and calf muscles (gastrocnemius and soleus).

Sesamoid bones are small bones that develop within a tendon, independent of the rest of the skeleton. They are located in the tendons that cover a joint, most commonly found under the head of the first metatarsal. Their purpose is to protect the tendon as it moves over the joint.

Task 20 • a) Name two of the main weight-bearing bones in the foot.
 b) What are the two main functions of the foot?
 c) To which bone and muscles is the Achilles tendon attached?

DISORDERS OF THE BONES AND JOINTS OF THE FEET:

Condition	Cause
Gout	Metabolic disorder. Excessive uric acid in the blood (forms crystals, causing inflammation)
	Arthritis
	Wear and tear on joints
	Metabolic factors
Osteoporosis	Ageing
	Menopause (reduced oestrogen)
	Poor diet (calcium deficiency)
	Hormonal disorders
	Prolonged immobility
	Hereditary condition
Fallen arches	Weakness or tearing of muscles or ligaments of foot
	Excess body weight
	Prolonged foot strain (standing or walking)
	Injury
	High-heeled shoes
	Malnutrition
Hammer toes	Abnormality of tendon
	Ill-fitting footwear
	Disease (e.g. arthritis)
	Hereditary condition
Heel spurs	Prolonged muscle or ligament strain
	Prolonged standing
	Prolonged wearing of improper shoes
	Inherited weakness

The feet

Chapter 9

THE SOLE

The sole of the foot is different to skin elsewhere on the body because it is thicker and contains no hair follicles or sebaceous glands.

Task 21 • a) How many bones are there in each foot?

b) Give two functions of the arches of the foot.

c) Name four of the bones that form the tarsus.

d)   i) What are sesamoid bones?

   ii) Where are they found in the foot?

  iii) What are their function?

Task 22 • a) Name six common disorders of the feet.

b) State two ways in which the skin on the sole of the foot is different from that elsewhere on the body.

CONDITIONS OF THE FEET

A reflexologist is not a trained chiropodist/podiatrist and therefore cannot be expected to give detailed advice on foot care or be able to treat foot conditions. However, the foot is the chosen point of access for the treatment and as such it is very important that a reflexologist can recognise common foot problems, so that the correct referral advice can be given. Many chiropodists/podiatrists are now also trained as reflexologists – an extra bonus to the client!

SOME COMMON FOOT DISORDERS

Name	Description	Causes
Callosities or Callus	An area of hard skin of fairly even thickness formed to protect the foot from pressure or friction	Ill-fitting shoes, uneven body weight or stretched ligaments in the foot. Treatment can involve paring away the thickened skin or wearing special padded insoles to ease the discomfort when wearing shoes

Name	Description	Causes
Corns	An area of callus where the pressure or friction is applied over a bony prominence or tendon. Excessive cell division in the skin then produces a conical mass of dead cells which is called a nucleus. This hard nucleus serves only to increase the original problem.	Ill-fitting shoes uneven body weight or stretched ligaments in the foot
Enlarged joint ('bunion') or Hallux valgus	A deformity where the big toe deviates towards the outside of the foot. The bones, ligaments, cartilage, tendons and sesamoids of the first metatarso-phalangeal joint also becomes displaced and the joint protrudes 	Caused mostly by ill-fitting shoes but can also be caused from inherited joint weakness, poor circulation or certain skin diseases. A bunion is often very painful and gentle handling is essential. Successfully treated, especially in the early stages before osteo-arthritis and ankylosis (stillness) occur. Surgery is the last, and not always satisfactory, resort

Name	Description	Causes
Verrucae (Plantar warts)	Highly vascular warts. Characteristics are the clear, circumscribed boundary and the dark dots formed by vascular tufts, which run through many verrucae. Some types disappear on their own, others reproduce asexually on the foot to form many (sometimes hundreds) 'daughter' verrucae, especially if the person's immunity is low. They can be extremely painful. Correct diagnosis may require microscopy, as many verrucae are masked by thick layers of callus	A viral infection which can be easily spread especially in summer and autumn when warm weather and barefoot activities coincide. Verrucae can be removed with the use of acid and weekly paring, or by cryosurgery (the use of cold or freezing in treatment). The latter can be painful. Verrucidal substances include banana 'pith', garlic, tea tree oil, thuja and lemon juice. Reflexologists must wash their hands after treating infected clients as verrucae can spread to hands and faces. The affected area should be avoided during treatment or covered

Name	Description	Causes
Ingrowing toenails	Inflammation (or sepsis) due to a spur of nail which pierces the flesh down the side of the nail	Often caused by poor nail cutting or pressure from shoes or a neighbouring toe. Treatment involves dealing with the infection, removal of the nail splinter and removal of the cause of the condition
Chilblain	Blood vessels contract causing the skin to go numb, red and swollen and itchy. The skin can also break	Poor circulation. Extreme reaction to cold. The condition is made worse with exposure to cold and damp
Athlete's foot (Tinea pedis)	Fungal condition at the base of or between the toes. It is shown as flaky, scaling skin often split between the toes, with an unpleasant smell	Fungal. Could be caused by allergic reaction. Warmth and moisture aggravate the condition. Treatment usually by anti-fungal creams or ointment. Avoid the area during the reflexology treatment

 Task 23 • a) Describe the condition commonly known as athlete's foot. Give a possible cause of such a condition.

b) i) What is the conventional treatment for athlete's foot?

ii) How would a reflexologist deal with this whilst working?

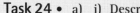

Task 24 •
a) i) Describe the condition known as a 'bunion'.
    ii) Give two possible causes of such a condition.
b) i) What is a skin callous?
    ii) Give two causes of such a condition.
c) Describe a possible treatment for:
    i) a bunion
    ii) a callous.

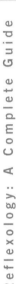

BACTERIAL INFECTIONS

A cut foot, ingrowing toenail, corn, splintered site etc. can easily become infected. Below are some of the terms to describe various degrees of severity.

Name	Description
Inflammation	The term to describe the response to damage. Featuring redness, warmth, swelling and pain with impaired function of the damaged area. Vast numbers of certain white blood cells mass at the site to fight the invading bacteria
Sepsis	Pus may build up or ooze from the wound
Lymphangitis	Faint red trails are seen on the inside of the leg (leading to behind the knee where the lymph nodes are). These are infected lymph vessels. The client may feel unwell, shivery, sweaty, feverish etc
Ulcer	Destruction of the skin involving DERMIS. Hard to heal
Cellulitis	Deeper tissues are concerned. Both muscles and bones may be affected. Suppuration (pus), fever and distress are evident.
Necrosis	Death of tissue or cells (in a small area)
Gangrene	Necrosis of a considerable mass of tissue. The area looks dark

As discussed in Chapter 8 reflexology should not be undertaken if the client has a severe bacterial infection.

The reflexologist can take a number of precautions to avoid contracting an infection whilst treating the foot, such as avoiding contact with the affected area or covering the infected area with a plaster. If you are concerned about the condition of a client's feet then suggest a check-up by a chiropodist/podiatrist or doctor before proceeding with the treatment.

CONDITIONS OF THE TOENAIL

Condition	Cause
Toenail infections	Bacteria or fungal infection
Avulsion (loss/removal of toenail)	Accident or injury
	Surgery
Club nail (Rams horn nail)	Systemic disease
	Neglect
	Injury
Calloused nail groove	Continued friction against nail plate
Brittle, ridged, concave nails	Iron deficiency anaemia
Inflammation of the cuticle	Frequent immersion in water

DIABETES MELLITUS

Diabetes Mellitus is caused by deficient or inadequate insulin production. Degenerative changes may occur in the ageing diabetic feet, which are of great importance to the reflexologist.

1. Ischaemia, reducing blood flow to the feet, will lead to damage to the nerve endings thereby causing numbness and loss of feeling (peripheral neuropathy). The diabetic may damage his/her foot without realising it.

2. White blood cells (defence) may become reduced in number or may become less effective at fighting infections.

3. As a result of lowered resistance to infection ulcers or even gangrene can quickly result.

To avoid risk of amputation early referral is essential.

STATES OR CONDITIONS OF THE FEET RESULTING FROM DIABETES MELLITUS

*   Loss of sensation (damage to nerve endings).

*   Brittle, easily cracked or damaged skin.

*   Danger of cuts or sores developing into ulceration or gangrene.

*   Poor circulation/reduced blood flow.

- Loss of flexibility/elasticity of skin.
- Excessive sweating.

- Reduced ability of skin to heal.
- Oedema.

In general there is a greater risk of infection developing because of changed cellular environment (excess blood sugar creates favourable conditions for bacterial growth).

106

Task 25 • a) Name four states or conditions of the feet that could result from diabetes mellitus.
　　　　　b) i) State which foot condition is infectious:
　　　　　　　　Corns　　Verrucae　　Eczema
　　　　　　ii) What precaution can be taken by the reflexologist to prevent contraction of the infection?
　　　　　c) Name two conditions affecting the toenail, and a possible cause for each.

CIRCULATORY CONDITIONS

During normal movement the calf muscles assist, by their pumping action, to squeeze the blood in the legs back to the heart, allowing fresh oxygenated blood to flow into the leg and foot. Several conditions can affect this normal function:

Condition	Description
Atheroma (atherosclerosis)	A very common form of arterial disease in which narrowing due to deposits of fatty material leads to diminution or failure of blood supply to various tissues
Ischaemia	Insufficient blood supply
Venous thrombosis	Blood clots in the veins are extremely serious. Thrombosis usually begins in deep veins of the calf and may be accompanied by pain. Its most serious complication is pulmonary embolism, which follows dislodgement of the thrombus shortly after it has formed. See Chapter 8 for more details.

Condition	Description
Varicose veins	Due to a failure of valves in the long saphenous vein. The back-pressure of blood stretches the walls of these veins which become flabby, like thin bags. Stagnation of blood in these veins can cause inflammation. They become dilated and tortuous. These veins may rupture causing severe haemorrhage which is controlled by raising the leg and applying pressure (with appropriate dressings).
Varicose eczema	Scaly eruption where the skin is pigmented (dusky red or mottled).
Phlebitis	Inflammation of a vein. Usually due to varicosity (in the legs). The vein, if accessible, is felt as a hard, tender cord over which the skin is hot and dusky in appearance. The inflammation causes roughening of the inner lining of the vein at the site of which blood may start to clot and thus the process of thrombosis develops. See Chapter 8 for more details.

CONDITIONS OF THE SWEAT GLANDS (FEET)

When sweating does not occur there must always be a suspicion of organic disease. Causes may include hypothalamic disease, diabetes, absence of sweat glands, eczema, psoriasis etc. Treatment will be directed towards the basic cause if possible. Failing this, and for use on clients who have dry and thickened skin, regular use of emollients such as a cream or lotion may reduce discomfort.

Sweaty feet can be helped with treatment by a chiropodist/podiatrist. Causes vary from adolescent nerves and hormonal imbalance to flat feet. There is often a family history of this problem. Regular washing and avoidance of restricted footwear are important.

Task 26 • a) What important function do the calf muscles perform in relation to the circulation in the foot?
b) Name three conditions that may involve a disorder of the circulation of the feet.

CHAPTER 10

Hand reflexology?

WHAT IS HAND REFLEXOLOGY

Hand reflexology follows exactly the same principals as foot reflexology. The human body is completely reflected in the hands in the same way as the feet. A point on the hand which relates to an area of the body is also called a reflex in the same way as a foot reflex.

By applying pressure to the reflex areas of the hands the reflexologist can locate blockages and imbalances of the zone pathways which, through treatment, can be corrected thus restoring the flow of the body's natural healing energies and aiding a return to good health.

Refer to Chapter 3 for an example hand reflexology sequence and illustrations of commonly taught reflex areas. It is usual for a full hand reflexology treatment to be completed in a shorter time than a foot treatment (approximately 30 minutes). There are a variety of hand reflexology charts available, however, it is best to refer to your preferred chart in order to learn the sequence and the location of reflex areas, but always be open to different approaches and techniques.

It is usual for most practising reflexologists to use the hand reflexes to supplement a foot treatment rather than give a whole hand treatment. In these instances a 'sequence' is not followed; instead, various reflex points are treated on the hand to supplement the work on the feet. This is not always the case, however, and other options are discussed below.

WHY USE HAND REFLEXOLOGY?

Hand reflexology can be given *instead* of a foot treatment for a variety of reasons:

- The foot is damaged or injured.
- The client feels the foot is too sensitive.
- The client does not want the foot to be treated.
- The foot is infected.
- The foot has been amputated.

- If access to the feet is too difficult.

- As a self-help treatment.

- When there is not enough time for a foot treatment.

- For demonstration purposes.

On some occasions it may also be helpful to give some hand reflexology (but not a *full* treatment):

- As homework for a client between treatments.

- As a self-help treatment.

- To reinforce reflex areas worked on the foot.

- For demonstration purposes.

- As a first-aid treatment.

It is also possible that a client may prefer to have a hand rather than a foot treatment:

- The client is embarrassed to show their feet.

- The client prefers the sensation of a hands treatment.

- A shorter time is more convenient.

- The foot-raised position is too uncomfortable.

- The client fears 'ticklish feet'.

Task 27 • a) Give two reasons why a client may prefer to have a hand reflexology treatment.
  b) Give three reasons why you might give a hand reflexology treatment instead of a foot reflexology treatment.
  c) Give two reasons why the use of some hand reflexology (as opposed to a full treatment) might be appropriate.

THE POSITIONS

The nature of a hand reflexology treatment requires the practitioner to adopt a position closer to the client. There are several possibilities:

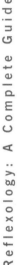

- sitting face to face, using a cushion as a support for the hand

- sitting at a bedside alongside the client

- sitting face to face with a table in between on which to support the hand

- sitting by the side of a couch or recliner

- sitting at a bedside facing the client.

The practitioner must be aware that because of the close nature of a hand reflexology treatment some clients may feel intimidated by the practitioner taking a position directly facing them as it may invade the client's personal space. It must also be remembered that some people consider their hands to be a more intimate area of the body than their feet!

A hand reflexology treatment differs from that of the feet in several ways:

- The skin on the hand is looser.

- The hand is floppier and less easy to control.

- The treatment is quicker to complete.

- The hands are easier to access.

- The reflex points take longer to respond (need to stay on point slightly longer).

- The abdominal area is much smaller.

Task 28 • a) Describe three possible positions of the client and practitioner during a hand reflexology treatment.
b) Describe three ways in which working on the hands differs from the feet.

SOME COMMON DISEASES AND CONDITIONS OF THE HANDS

Condition	Description
Raynauds disease	Blood vessel disorder causing small arteries to fingers to contract suddenly, cutting off blood flow to the fingers
Eczema	Inflammation of the skin causing itching and sometimes scaling and blisters

Condition	Description
Osteoporosis	Loss of protein tissue from bone causing it to become brittle and easily fractured
Rheumatoid arthritis	Joint inflammation causing pain, swelling and stiffness in the joints of fingers and toes
Osteoarthritis	Degeneration of the cartilage that lines the joints
Carpal tunnel syndrome	Pressure on the median nerve where it passes into the hand, causing numbness, tingling and pain in the thumb, index and middle fingers
Ganglion	A cystic swelling associated with the sheath of a tendon. Usually pea size but can be bigger
Warts	A harmless growth on skin. Contagious
Contact dermatitis	A skin reaction to various substances (varies according to the individual). Shown as bubbles on the hands that can become itchy and weepy
RSI (Repetitive Strain Injury)	The inflammation of wrist, finger or thumb joints due to constantly repeating particular movements of the hands
Chilblain	Extreme reaction to cold. Blood vessels contract causing the skin to go numb, red and swollen and itchy. The skin can also break. The condition is made worse by exposure to cold and damp
Calluses	Area of thickened skin caused by regular or prolonged pressure or friction

 Task 29 • a) List four diseases or conditions that can be found on the hands.
b) What is carpal tunnel syndrome and what are the symptoms?

CHAPTER 11

Client consultation

KEEPING RECORDS OF TREATMENT

Apart from the reflexology treatment, taking a client's personal and treatment details is an important factor in gaining an understanding of both the client and their state of health. The reflexologist should keep the following records:

An initial client consultation card	Records a client's personal details, such as name and address. It should also detail medical history and the reason for seeking treatment
A treatment card	Records each treatment given to the client. Details should include date of treatment, sensitive reflex points and comments made by the client
A case history	Records the 'story' of a group of treatments. It summarises a client's general progress through a set of treatments and draws a conclusion at the end as to the benefits of the sessions. A case history is usually required for examinations but is also useful once qualified as it helps draw conclusions to treatments.

THE INITIAL CLIENT CONSULTATION CARD

The format of the initial client consultation card is a matter for each practitioner. As a minimum it should contain the following client information:

1. Name, address and contact numbers

2. Doctor's name, address and contact number

3. Date of birth. Medical history: major operations, current and past medical conditions. Family medical history (hereditary conditions)

4. Presence of any contraindications

5. Reasons for seeking treatment

6. Lifestyle factors, for example occupation, leisure activities, smoking etc.

The initial client consultation card shown in Figure 12 is an example; you can use your preferred format with information shown in an order that best makes sense to you.

The initial consultation enables the practitioner to gain some indication of the client's overall condition. Completing a consultation card is important because it:

- checks for contraindications that show when caution may be appropriate during treatment

- gathers past medical history and gives information on current conditions

- establishes whether a referral is necessary

- gives an insight into lifestyle and thus indicates possible stress and emotional factors

- provides first basis for a treatment plan or focus of treatment

- establishes an overall picture of the individual

- collects administrative information such as name, address, doctor etc.

- may help to support findings during the reflexology treatment.

Task 30 • When seeing a client for the first time it is important to take an initial consultation. List what you consider to be five important questions that should be asked and recorded before the first treatment begins.

THE TREATMENT CARD

The format of the treatment card is a matter for each practitioner. As a minimum it should contain the following information:

- Date of the treatment.

- Client's feedback since last treatment.

- Sensitive reflex areas.

- Reflex areas given extra attention.

PRACTITIONER'S NAME:

CLIENT CONSULTATION

NAME _____

ADDRESS _____

OCCUPATION _____

TEL. No. _____ DATE OF BIRTH ___/___/___

Dr's Name _____ Address _____

Tel. No. _____

REFERRED BY:

MEDICATION: (Birth pill, Hormone therapy, Prescription drugs etc):

OPERATIONS/X-RAY:

ACCIDENTS:

INFECTIONS:

OTHER COMPLAINTS: (Allergies, Migraine, Blood pressure, Bladder, Heart, Kidneys, Skin, Epilepsy, Diabetes, Family history etc):

Check for contraindications (Thrombosis, Phlebitis etc) CHECKED:
☐ tick if none or detail contraindications:

STRESSES

ORTHODOX
TREATMENT:

/over...

Principal complaint/s:

Original onset:

Symptoms:

Part of body affected:

Frequency:

Previous treatments:

What makes it worse and/or better:

Is there anything else I need to know:

First treatment date:

FEET OBSERVATION

Condition of feet:

PATIENT'S SIGNATURE	PRACTITIONER'S SIGNATURE

Figure 12. Sample client consultation card

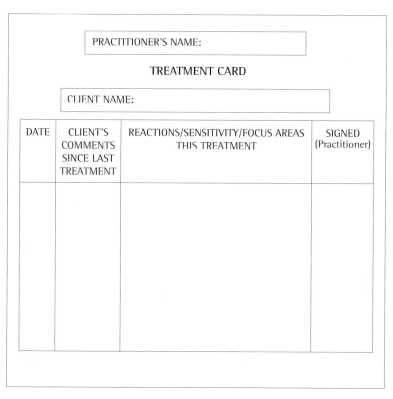

Figure 13 Sample client treatment card

The treatment card shown in Figure 13 is an example; use a format with the information shown in an order that best makes sense to you.

The treatment card must be completed because it:

- records the date of each treatment session

- records client reactions/sensitive reflex points

- records changes in treatment emphasis

- keeps account of the effectiveness of the overall treatment process

- is a requirement of most practitioner insurance policies

- helps the practitioner to formulate a continuing holistic treatment pattern.

The treatment card is a very important tool for helping the practitioner to remember previous treatments and thus form an effective treatment process. The practitioner can look back on previous treatments recorded on the card and assess the effectiveness of the treatment and any changes in sensitive reflex points. It also provides a valuable point of reference for treating other clients with similar conditions.

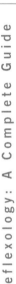
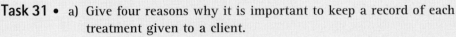

Task 31 • a) Give four reasons why it is important to keep a record of each treatment given to a client.
  b) Name what you consider to be four of the most important items to include when completing your record of a treatment session.

CASE HISTORY

A case history is a useful summary of a complete course of reflexology treatments and is kept for the following reasons:

- It illustrates the effectiveness of an overall set of treatments.

- It helps with practitioner's self-development.

- It serves as a useful reference for treating clients with similar presenting problems.

- It may be useful for general research data.

RECOMMENDED PROCEDURE

1. Set out the initial problem area and initial observations.

2. Describe treatment given (e.g. if you have concentrated on particular areas due to the presenting problem).

3. Describe any links between sensitive areas and the main presenting problems.

4. Detail any progression from the main presenting problem i.e. other problems become apparent.

5. Detail any advice given.

6. Detail the improvement made and client comments as to the effectiveness of the treatment.

7. Summary.

8. Final comments.

9. Your thoughts.

Note: The length of the case history is not important – it is the content that matters. As a guide the average case history is about one side of A4 although it could be less – the maximum should be two sides of A4 unless in exceptional circumstances. Obviously it is not possible to complete a case history until a course of treatments has been completed – usually between five and ten treatments.

EXAMINATION REQUIREMENTS: RECORD CARDS AND CASE HISTORIES

For students who are sitting a formal reflexology exam it is normal to show proof of reflexology treatments. It is the evidence of the recording of the initial consultation, subsequent treatments and a case history that is important rather than the exact format of the information itself. You must repeat your preferred format for each client so you can demonstrate a consistent and organised approach.

INSURANCE AND DISCLAIMERS

Although reflexology is a very safe form of treatment it is recommended that students join a reflexology organisation such as The Association of Reflexologists as a student member, ensuring this includes student insurance. Insurance will protect you from any possible claims that may be made by clients (see Chapters 22–29 for more details). While training, some practitioners may also prefer to request their clients to sign a disclaimer. This is a document that clearly sets out the position of both the client and the practitioner. An example of a disclaimer could be:

I understand that the below signed is a student of reflexology. I consent to becoming a case study for reflexology treatments, and understand that the treatment is not from a qualified practitioner, and that I can make no claim whatsoever against the student arising from the administering of the treatment as it is administered for study purposes only and forms part of the practice work required towards completion of the course. I also understand that notes from the session(s) may be made available to a third party for assessment of the students competence.

Signed by student _____ Print name_____

Signed by client/case study _____ Print name_____

Date_____.

CONFIDENTIALITY

It is very important that client consultation and treatment cards remain confidential. As a practitioner you are in a position of trust and responsibility. Let your clients know that you treat your sessions as confidential and that any information given will be treated as such. In order for the records to remain confidential you must take the following action:

- Keep them in a secure place, preferably a locked cabinet.

- Do not allow others access to your client records.

- Do not discuss personal details of your clients to others. You may, of course, need to discuss details of various clients' conditions with other healthcare professionals or tutors or for research projects. In these cases any of the client's identifying details such as name, address and doctor should be withheld. All other details that do not personally identify the client can then be presented anonymously, thus protecting the client's confidentiality.

 Task 32 • Describe two ways in which you would ensure that client records remained confidential.

CHAPTER 12

Observation of the client and their feet – and what it can tell you

As well as the initial consultation and the treatment itself, there are two other factors that are useful for the reflexologist in establishing a picture of the individual and thus helping with a treatment pattern:

- non-verbal communication

- observation of the feet.

NON-VERBAL COMMUNICATION

It is said that only 7 per cent of communication is verbal therefore it is wise to be alert to any non-verbal signs given by the client. In practice this means using both our common sense and that feeling of intuition that we all have about the nature of others.

It is also often said that we form judgements about people within the first 30 seconds of meeting them – you must not fall into this trap as a practitioner. Do not allow any initial thoughts and feelings you have towards a client to become a rigid judgement, for example just because someone is wearing a dirty T-shirt it does not necessarily mean they have hygiene problems or are sleeping rough – it could just be that their washing machine is broken. In other words, use the non-verbal information given to you by the client, but only in terms of helping you towards an understanding of their nature and therefore helping to form a treatment that is appropriate to them. Use it in conjunction with all the other assessment criteria available to you – not as a one-stop judgement and solution.

For example a male client turns up ten minutes late, in a smart business suit, and deep in a confrontational conversation on a mobile phone. This may give you a clue to his occupation, his lifestyle and even his opinions and politics. It does not necessarily mean that your observations are correct – he may not be a stressed-out business man who needs relaxation and sleep-inducing treatments; he may be enjoying his work and wanting more energy to tackle his exciting tasks. This may not become apparent until after the initial consultation or during the treatment itself. In other words be open to the clues presented to you but do not rely upon them!

Further observation of the client will reveal the following non-verbal clues:

- Physical disability
- Ease of movement
- Breathing
- Posture

- Skin colour and texture
- Weight
- Eye contact (or lack of it)
- Condition of skin, hair, eyes

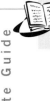

Task 33 • As reflexologists, apart from looking at the feet, we should observe our clients for other clues to their general condition and state of well being. List four of the clues we could look for.

OBSERVATION OF THE FEET

Once the initial consultation has been taken it is important to take a good look at the feet before starting the actual treatment. By observing the feet the practitioner can add another layer of information about the client. The observation can take place during the opening movements of the sequence. Observations of the feet may yield some of the following:

Dry rough skin	Scars	Bunions
Skin colour	Freckles	Corns
Peeling skin	Wrinkles and folds	Moles
Smell	Vein disorders	Hair growth
Sweating or moisture	Lines and grooves	Cracks
Calluses	Swollen areas	Ulcers/sores
Puffiness	Eczema	Texture
Flakiness	Athlete's foot	Nail condition
Structure/deformity	Warts or verrucae	Toe shape/position

Bone growth

It is useful to record your observations of the feet on the client consultation or treatment card. If any of the above are present it does not necessarily mean anything in itself but may give an indication of the client's state of health. It should be viewed together with other information taken in the initial consultation and from reactions to the reflex treatment itself before arriving at a conclusion. For this reason observations of the condition of the feet are often known as 'indicators'. Below are some suggested examples of how indicators could be incorporated into a treatment. The important thing to remember about these examples is that, depending on the overall information available, a different treatment plan can be arrived at for the same physical indicator:

Indicator	Client information from initial consultation	Reflex information	Treatment plan
Bunion – big toe	None specific to indicator	Sensitive on bunion area	No specific links – treat lightly on bunion areas
Bunion – big toe	Job involves standing for long periods. Wears tight shoes	Sensitive on bunion area and red, sore areas around heel	Extra work to relax and stretch the feet. Extra work to thymus and adrenal reflexes to aid healing and pain relief. Advise better fitting shoes!
Wet, perspiring feet	None relevant	Sensitive thyroid and thymus	Extra work to endocrine system for hormonal balance. Check with client for further information relating to hormonal imbalance i.e. energy levels, sleep patterns etc.
Wet, perspiring feet	Nervous of new situations. Feels stressed with current work pressures.	Crystals around head and neck. Sensitive solar plexus and diaphragm	Extra relaxation techniques to help stress levels. More work on diaphragm and solar plexus. Extra rotations and stretching on head and neck

Task 34 • As reflexologists we may look for indicators to a client's health by observing the condition of the feet or noting the differences between the feet.

 a) List eight of these indicators that may be present on a visual examination of a client's feet.

 b) Give two possible assessments that could be made from the observation that your client has very wet, perspiring feet.

OTHER LINKS

It is also possible that observations of physical indicators on the feet are linked directly to the body *through the reflex areas* on which they appear. Once again this link is to be treated with caution and other evidence should be taken into account before drawing a definite conclusion. Some possible example links are:

Physical indicator	Possible reflex link
Fallen arch	Occurs on the spinal reflexes therefore be aware of possible spinal problems/back aches/postural difficulties
Callusing on top of toes	Occurs on sinus reflexes therefore possible sinus problems. Congestion of nasal passages. Polyps or excessive mucous
Dry, rough skin around heel	Occurs on lower back/sciatic/sacrum reflex areas therefore possible lower back problems or sciatica. Possible pelvis problems
Bunion on big toe	Occurs on neck and thyroid reflex areas therefore possible neck problems or hormonal imbalance
Ingrowing toenail	Occurs on head and neck reflex areas therefore possible link to headaches, migraine and stress

Task 35 • Give a possible problem each of the following conditions might indicate in the body:
   a) Ingrowing toenail
   b) Fallen longitudinal arch
   c) Bunion.

CHAPTER 13

Assessing the client's treatment needs – three paths to understanding

Once a reflexologist learns and is comfortable with a treatment sequence it is then time to apply thought to the actual treatment process for each client. However competent your treatment, it cannot be applied mechanically in the same way to every client, as each client will have their own needs from the treatment. How do we find out what each client needs from a treatment and how do we best 'gather evidence' to assist the treatment process?

We have seen from the previous chapters that the reflexologist needs to build up a whole picture of the individual in order to give as complete a treatment as possible. A reflexologist must develop the ability to touch a person and to react to his or her actual state, to understand the patterns, systems and processes that brought that person to their present condition.

The previous chapters have already described the three ways a practitioner can gather evidence towards a client's treatment requirements:

1. Initial client consultation: Questioning and listening to the individual. The recalling of things past (medical history, profession, nutrition habits, stress/emotional factors, present conditions).

2. Observation of client and visual check of feet: Possible indications: dry rough skin, bunions, corns, warts, athlete's foot, eczema, change of skin colour, skin peel, bone structure, shape of toes, shape of arches, swollen areas, perspiration of feet, weight distribution, comparison between feet.

3. The reflexology treatment: Information gathered through the touching process of the reflex treatment e.g.: crystalline deposits, muscular tone, lumps and/or nodes in the muscles, painful points or areas, sensitivity or loss of sensitivity in points, areas that feel swollen, lack or excess of movements in feet joints, change of temperature between areas of the foot or between the feet.

The above diagnostic information gathering can be viewed as the three paths to understanding.

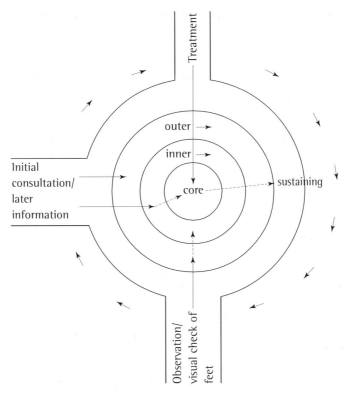

Figure 14 The three paths to understanding

 Task 36 • List three basic ways a reflexologist assesses the condition and treatment needs of a client.

As Figure 14 demonstrates, the treatment process follows the above paths towards a deeper understanding and treatment of the individual. In most clients the paths lead to the 'core' treatment and healing in the following way:

1. **The initial consultation**

• Gives an indication of the basic path of treatment to be followed.

• Alerts the practitioner to possible contraindications and relevant medical history including distant and recent conditions etc.

• Outlines client expectation and begins client/practitioner relationship.

2. **The outer treatments**

• The initial treatments serve to further establish the treatment pattern and give the practitioner initial detailed knowledge of presenting areas of sensitivity.

- Help to stimulate the flow of energies and begin to 'treat as a whole'.

3. **The core treatments**

- Throughout the following treatments an interchange of information takes place between the practitioner and client which helps to establish the emphasis of treatment.

- The practitioner is able to re-evaluate the treatment at each session by listening to client reactions to treatment and noting changes in their feet. An 'opening up' process will be established with further information given by the client, helping the practitioner to focus on underlying problems. The practitioner will be able to identify basic tendencies and areas of vulnerability, specific to the person, and formulate a whole approach to treatment.

4. **The sustaining treatments**

- This stage is reached from the core treatments only when continual reassessment from the practitioner indicates that the desired effect has been reached.

- These treatments are less regular and serve to retain the benefits of the whole process. They provide reassurance to the client and may also alert the reflexologist to new presenting problems.

5. **In conclusion:** The treatment process can be likened to the peeling of an onion – getting closer to the core layer by layer. The more skilled a reflexologist becomes in gathering and assessing information from the client the better he or she can view the client's development and uncompleted processes which are at their very beginning and may not show on the surface.

CAUTION!

It is not within the realms of reflexology to diagnose in a conventional sense nor should the practitioner claim the ability to achieve this. It is valid, however, for the practitioner to examine, assess, understand and unravel the complexities of the individual body receiving treatment in order to attempt the best possible treatment. In this sense diagnostic skills are a vital part of the reflexologist's skills.

Guidance on how to view diagnosis within the context of a reflexology treatment can be found in the documents below:

Paragraph 2.15 of the 'Code of Conduct and Guidance to Practitioners' issued by The National Consultative Council for Alternative and Complementary Medicine states:

'Practitioners must never give a **medical** diagnosis to a patient/client in any circumstances; this is the responsibility of a registered medical practitioner. However, many practitioners have a 'gift' of diagnosis and of discovering dysfunctions in the physical, emotional, mental and spiritual aspects and in this case the practitioner may make mention of any disorder which he may discover, and advise the patient/client to see the doctor for a **medical** diagnosis and record this action.'

Paragraph 2 section 4 of The Association of Reflexologists 'Code of Practice and Ethics' states:

'Members should not diagnose a medical condition, prescribe or treat a specific ailment in connection with reflexology treatment or use implements.'

CHAPTER 14

Arrangement of treatment sessions and other treatment practicalities

Having the knowledge of how reflexology works, applying it and achieving an understanding of the client's condition will help the practitioner only once the actual practicalities of the treatment sessions are understood. It is very important that a professional approach to these practicalities is taken at all times. A professional approach is necessary for the confidence of both the practitioner and the client. This chapter is intended to deal only with the professional approach needed during the actual treatment sessions. Further aspects of running a reflexology practice will be discussed in Chapters 22–29.

The practicalities of treatment can be broken down into the following main activities:

- **P**repare
- **R**eceive   and
- **E**ngage

- **A**ssure
- **F**ollow-up
- **T**erminate

Remember this as PRE and AFT treatment. The activities can be explained as follows:

PREPARE

Activity	Reason
Allow a break between clients	To 'reset' treatment area (new couch paper etc).
	For practitioner to rest.
	In case treatment overruns
Set answering machine/turn phone off	Client and practitioner not disturbed.
	No distractions to treatment
Client records	Get new client form and pen
	or
	Read existing consultation and treatment card to refresh memory

RECEIVE

Activity	Reason
First-time client	
Shake hands, introduce yourself and give your qualifications and brief background	Instils confidence in the client, is a professional approach for practitioner. Begins client/practitioner relationship
First-time client	
Explain what reflexology is	Puts client at ease, is a professional approach for practitioner
First-time client	
Briefly explain what the treatment procedure involves i.e. a) consultation form (including contraindications etc) b) recline and remove shoes and socks c) pressure to feet d) some areas may feel slight discomfort e) you may feel like closing your eyes and relaxing f) can last between 50 minutes and 1 hour	Puts clients at ease. Outlines the role and expectations of client and practitioner. Highlights that consultation is confidential
Existing client	
Greet using their name	Puts client at ease, makes them feel like an individual
Existing client	
Enquire progress since last session	Helps practitioner evaluate treatments, makes client feel valued
Follow up any relevant treatment issues	Helps practitioner evaluate treatments and works towards the treatments paths and core treatments (see Chapter 13)

ENGAGE

Activity	Reason
Remove shoes and socks	Comfort of client/practitioner access to feet for observation and treatment
Help client onto couch/chair	Comfort of client, safety of client
Feet raised, with knees supported	Comfort of client and access for practitioner to treat
Head raised within view of practitioner, neck and shoulders supported	Comfort and reassurance of client. Practitioner can view client reactions and interact with client if necessary
Practitioner seated with client's feet at chest level	Comfort of practitioner, optimum view of feet for treatment
Practitioner with back straight on height adjustable stool (with wheels if possible)	Comfort of practitioner. Ability of practitioner to move easily to best treatment position
Practitioner with clipboard or small side table	Enables practitioner to have treatment card to hand in order to record client reactions, and thus assess and evaluate treatment process

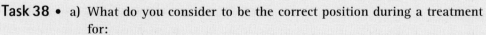

Task 37 • a) List four points you would make to a new or prospective client when describing to them what to expect during a treatment session.
   b) Give a possible reason behind each of the statements listed below:
      i) It is a good idea to arrange treatment sessions with a break between clients.
      ii) I have a height-adjustable stool with wheels from which to treat.
      iii) I never answer the telephone during a treatment.
      iv) I like to help clients on and off the treatment chair or couch.

Task 38 • a) What do you consider to be the correct position during a treatment for:
      i) The client
      ii) The therapist?
Give your reasons.

Then, following the actual treatment:

ASSURE

Activity	Reason
Check client is fully awake	Establishes client can be moved
Help client from chair/couch	For safety and comfort of client
Reinstate that the treatment will help the body's healing mechanisms, and that all information recorded is confidential	Reassures client that the treatment can help them. Emphasises the client/practitioner relationship and builds trust between both parties.
Mention that sensitive reflex areas or areas that hurt are a normal part of the treatment and that: a) it helps the practitioner to treat and balance the body b) it is an indication of the body responding to the treatment c) it gives a general indication as to the body's overall state of health and *does not* mean any one organ is 'damaged'.	Reassures client that their reactions are not extreme. Prevents client concern about a particular sensitive reflex. Helps build confidence in the treatment procedure

FOLLOW-UP

Activity	Reason
Number of treatments Mention that each client is different, depending on: a) reason for treatment b) response to treatment c) the particular condition(s)	Gives client an idea of the time, frequency and financial commitment required.

Reflexology: A Complete Guide

Activity	Reason
d) how long the condition(s) has been present e) feedback from future treatments f) client's age and financial circumstances Give an indication of the average number of treatments (e.g. 5–10, weekly)	

Length of treatments

You may wish to vary the length of the treatment taking into account some of the following factors: a) age of client b) health condition c) sensitivity of reflexes d) financial circumstances of client If this is relevant, then inform the client of your reasons for varying the length of treatment.	Reassures client about future length of treatments. Client feels treated as an individual. Builds client/practitioner relationship

Reactions to treatment

Mention some of the common reactions to treatment for example: a) feeling tired b) feeling more energetic c) increase in urination/sweating d) temporary worsening of symptoms e) headaches f) thirst.	Gives client reassurance that reactions are part of the treatment process. Demonstrates that the practitioner has experience of the treatment process.

Activity	Reason
Explain reactions are part of the treatment process and are a sign of the body working to heal itself and possibly rid itself of toxins	Gives client reassurance that reactions are part of the treatment process

Aftercare advice

Activity	Reason
Give some general advice that will help the client to take full advantage of the treatment: a) be careful if driving home b) drink plenty of water c) avoid a heavy meal or alcohol for the rest of the day d) take some rest if you start to feel tired	Client begins to take some responsibility for the treatment process (see 'Holistic Approach' in Chapter 19). Demonstrates experience of practitioner

Self-treatment

Activity	Reason
It may be appropriate, in certain cases, to demonstrate one or two reflex points on the hands or feet (hands are usually easier as they are more accessible to the client). Explain that this can help with the healing process	Client begins to take some responsibility for the treatment process. May help accelerate the healing process. Demonstrates the experience of the practitioner. **Note:** Self-treatment has its advantages: a) no cost to client b) can be undertaken at a time convenient to client c) maintains progress between treatments d) good for emergency or first-aid situations But it also has disadvantages: a) can be uncomfortable

Activity	Reason
	b) does not have practitioner's trained knowledge
	c) relies upon client remembering!

TERMINATE

Activity	Reason
Arrange date of next appointment	To continue the treatment process and commit the client to taking part in their own health care
Give a card with your contact details (name, address, telephone number) and date of next appointment	Reminds client of practitioner's details should they need to contact before the next appointment. Reminds client of next appointment date, minimising chances of client not returning
Thank them for having reflexology and for continuing their treatment. Shake hands and escort them from the treatment room	Client feels valued. Demonstrates client's treatment time has ended

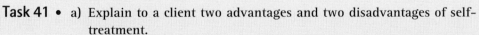

Task 39 • a) Detail two responses you could give if a client asked, 'Why does that point hurt?'
  b) Describe four points you would make to a client when giving your aftercare advice at the end of a treatment

Task 40 • a) When deciding on the number and regularity of treatments for a client, give two factors you would take into consideration.
  b) Give two factors which might influence the length of a treatment session.

Task 41 • a) Explain to a client two advantages and two disadvantages of self-treatment.
  b) Give a possible reason behind each of the statements listed below:
   i) I always give my clients a card with the date and time of their next treatment.
   ii) I like to help clients on and off the treatment chair or couch.

Task 42 • a) List four common reactions a client may experience after a reflexology treatment.

b) Give three possible reasons why a client may have a reaction after treatment.

CHAPTER 15

Other therapies and referrals

The reflexology practitioner must only give advice relating to the reflexology treatment. It is very important that no advice is given that is beyond the competence of the reflexologist. For example it would not be appropriate to give dietary or vitamin advice unless qualified to do so. In the same way it would not be appropriate to practise other therapies such as aromatherapy or massage on a reflexology client. The practitioner should not use or give advice on other therapies unless qualified to do so, and if qualified it should be made clear that they do not form part of the reflexology treatment.

The reflexologist does, however, work within the complementary therapy field and as such should be aware of other complementary therapies. We saw in Chapter 4 that:

'Reflexology is a form of complementary therapy. This means it can be used by itself or together with other forms of complementary or orthodox/allopathic treatment. It is not an alternative to medical treatment nor is it a way of diagnosing ailments or providing specific cures. It is a therapy that helps to release a client's own healing potential.'

An awareness of other therapies is essential for three main reasons:

1. Clients may have had other therapies before reflexology. It is important for the reflexologist to have a basic understanding of what is involved in other treatments, as it may have a bearing on the condition and future treatment of the client. It may also be considered unprofessional by the client if his/her reflexologist does not have a least a basic grasp of the other main complementary therapies.

2. Understanding the work of colleagues within the complementary therapy professions should work reciprocally. It may bring clients to you from colleagues who understand reflexology in the same way you understand their therapy.

3. It is part of the holistic philosophy (see later chapters).

OTHER COMPLEMENTARY THERAPIES

ACUPUNCTURE

This is a technique in which needles are used to puncture the skin at defined points along the body to restore the 'chi' energy.

There are around 800 points on the body which join up to form 12 major meridians. There is a pulse for each meridian and 28 qualities that can be recognised from the pulses.

AROMATHERAPY

This is the use of essential oils or aromatic essences of plants, which are applied through massage, used as inhalants or in baths or, rarely, ingested. In massage the essential oils are mixed with a base solution such as grapeseed oil. The oils penetrate the skin and, via the extra-cellular fluids, reach the blood and lymph from where they can be carried in the circulation to the organs.

BACH FLOWER REMEDIES

These are prepared from flowering wild plants, bushes and trees. They are not used directly for physical complaints but for the sufferers of worry, apprehension, irritability etc., because these states of mind or moods hinder the recovery of health and are regarded as the primary cause of sickness and disease.

The system was devised by Edward Bach, a Harley Street doctor and consultant. There are 38 Bach Flower remedies to cover all known negative states of mind, from apprehension to despondency and loneliness. The remedies are taken orally in an alcohol base.

CHIROPRACTIC

Chiropractors are specialists in the diagnosis and treatment of mechanical disorders of the joints, particularly of the spine, and their effects on the nervous system. X-rays are often used in diagnosis and a chiropractor carries out treatment by specific manipulation.

HOMOEOPATHY

A system of medicine developed from the natural law of *Similia similibus curantur* – like should be cured with like. This means that a substance or preparation which can cause a group of symptoms, whether physical, emotional or behavioural, in the healthy, can also cure similar groups of symptoms when they appear in the sick.

Samuel Hahnemann was the founder of homoeopathy in the late eighteenth century. Remedies are prepared from homoeopathic tinctures by a special process known as succussion. Each stage of succussion increases the potency which is given a number and a letter, such as 200C.

The more the remedy is diluted the stronger it gets. The remedies are usually taken in tablet form but are also available as ointments or tinctures.

MASSAGE

Massage is applied to the soft tissues of the body – the muscles and ligaments – but this also has a resulting beneficial effect on the nervous and circulatory systems.

NUTRITION

Food is the fuel of the body. The kind of food eaten can affect the processes of growth, repair and energy.

Nutritionists give advice on correct dietary requirements, which vary from person to person depending on their lifestyle, size, age, sex or weight etc. The aim is to improve the body's internal status for the prevention and curing of disease.

OSTEOPATHY

Osteopaths diagnose the body's misalignments by a method of sensitive touch and by observing the body's natural stance, appearance and posture. They aim to restore the body to its natural structural pattern by using manipulative techniques, high velocity thrusts and soft tissue work.

Cranial osteopathy is a gentle form of treatment to the head, and sometimes the body. The skull is made up of 22 bones joined together by hairline joints called sutures. The cranial technique gently manipulates the cranial bones to relieve pressure and produce a slight movement of the sutures.

PSYCHOTHERAPY

Psychotherapy aims to help a person to reconnect to their own source of healing energy and guidance. 'Psyche' from the Greek 'Psuche', meaning soul, has come to mean mind and soul in the modern interpretation. There are many approaches and techniques used in psychotherapy including talking through life situations, techniques for bringing through new insights and dreams, guided imagery, relaxation and creative expression. Work on the physical body may also play a part in the overall process.

Psychotherapy aims to enable individuals to find their own solutions in life and to deepen their self-understanding through exploring their feelings and attitudes in a non-judgemental way.

SHIATSU

Siatsu is a traditional Japanese healing therapy. It is used to rejuvenate the mind and body by stimulating points along the meridians. The hands, elbows, knees and feet are employed to apply pressure to the body.

There are many other therapies that could be considered complementary. Those listed above are believed by the author to be the most widely used therapies. Other loosely related therapies are Autogenics, Neuro-linguistic Programming and Reichian Therapy.

 Task 43 • **Name four other complementary therapies that might help a client with back pain. Give a brief description of each therapy.**

REFERRAL TO OTHER COMPLEMENTARY PRACTITIONERS

As mentioned earlier in the chapter, reflexologists must stay within the limits of their therapy training and experience. If it is the practitioner's judgement that a client could benefit from another form of therapy then it is acceptable to express your opinion, and explain the possible alternatives to the client. This must not be in a prescriptive way, but rather as a general comment. For example consider these two statements:

1. 'As you mentioned during your last treatment, your back is less painful but still very uncomfortable. I am sure reflexology is helping the body to deal with the problem, but have you thought about also seeing a chiropractor? It won't interfere with the reflexology treatment and I have heard that it can produce some good results with back problems.'

and

2. 'Your back is still very bad. You must see a chiropractor as soon as possible and tell him that the problems are between lumbar 3 and 5. Also take three analgesics a day'.

Statement (1) is acceptable because it provides some general guidance in line with the complementary philosophy but is clearly an expression of the practitioner's opinion, rather than a prescriptive, diagnostic statement.

Statement (2) is not acceptable because it appears to be a prescriptive statement containing diagnostic advice outside the practitioner's qualified experience.

A client may benefit from another form of complementary therapy for the following reasons:

- Many and complex symptoms would benefit from another approach.

- Client is not responding to reflexology.

- Reflexology is contraindicated (see Chapter 8).

- Reflexologist feels the condition is outside his/her ability as a practitioner.

RECOMMENDATIONS

If a client asks your advice in recommending another complementary practitioner, it would be helpful to suggest that the client uses the following 'get to know your therapist' checklist:

- What is the name of your qualification?

- Do you have insurance to practise?

- How long was your training course?

- How long have you been qualified?

- Do you belong to any professional organisations?

- Can the treatment help me?

This promotes the professionalism of complementary practitioners, all of whom should be happy to answer the above questions, if they have a satisfactory level of training and competence. The potential client will also feel more secure when receiving satisfactory answers from the therapist. The more the public are encouraged to ask the above questions, the more genuinely competent complementary practitioners will become identifiable.

> **Task 44** • a) Give two reasons why you might consider referring a client to another complementary health practitioner, apart from a reflexologist.
> b) Compile a list of four questions that, in your opinion, a prospective client should ask any complementary practitioner to establish their credentials and suitability before deciding upon treatment.

REFERRAL TO GP/DOCTOR

Care should be taken when suggesting that a client visits their GP/Doctor, as it may cause undue distress and worry. A practitioner should consider referral to a doctor when:

A   A client expresses concerns about a health problem. For example a client may mention that a mole has become darker and bigger since their last visit, and asks for your advice. This is not a problem reported to you during the initial consultation. A suggested response could be, 'I am not a doctor but I suggest that if you are concerned about the mole, you make an appointment with your doctor, as they are best qualified to give you medical advice.'

B   The client has a serious medical condition not yet seen by a doctor. A client may mention a serious medical condition during the initial consultation or during later treatments. If this condition has not yet received medical treatment then the practitioner must refer the client to a doctor.

C   The client has a medical condition the practitioner feels *should* be seen by a doctor. A client may not mention a serious medical condition but it may become evident to the practitioner. Without alarming the client the practitioner should suggest a visit to the GP/Doctor. For example: 'I have noticed a lump on your leg that has not gone away since the first treatment – I'm sure its nothing to worry about, but I think it would be worth letting your doctor take a look, because I am not medically qualified to investigate it.'

Alternatively, the appearance of symptoms that may indicate a medical problem should also be referred to a doctor. For example: 'You have said that you get severe stomach pains nearly every day and sometimes feel very dizzy. I am not a doctor but I suggest

that you visit your doctor so that you can find out what might be causing the problem.
I can, of course, give you treatments once you have checked with your doctor and
he/she is happy for you to continue with reflexology.'

Circumstances such as the above are rare occurrences, but it is essential that the practitioner
is aware of their duty of referral. When a practitioner suggests referral to a doctor it should
be recorded on the client treatment form. If a client refuses to see their doctor the
individual practitioner must decide whether or not to continue to treat the client. If a
practitioner continues to treat then a note of client refusal to see a doctor must be
recorded on the client treatment form. It is also advisable to get the client to sign a note to
this effect: 'I was advised on (date) by my reflexology practitioner to see a doctor for a
medical diagnosis. I have decided not to consult a doctor and to continue with the
reflexology treatments.'

Important note: the above refers to adult clients. Separate laws govern the treatment of
children. This will be discussed further in Section 4.

 Task 45 • State two circumstances when you would ask a client to consult their GP
or other medical professional.

CHAPTER 16

Treating common ailments

As discussed in previous chapters the paths to understanding give the reflexologist an insight into the treatment needs of the individual. While each client must make the journey along the treatment paths there are some common ailments that can present themselves in all clients. This is not to say that there are not other underlying causes or treatment plans to be formulated but that, at the same time, the presenting condition can be treated with emphasis on the reflex points.

COMMON AILMENTS WITH SUGGESTED EMPHASIS FOR TREATMENT

ADDICTION	Key reflex	Other reflex areas and reason
Addiction can affect people with an addictive personality. It can manifest as addictions to almost anything or several things at the same time.	*Pituitary/pineal/ hypothalamus* To balance the endocrine system, equalise mood swings, instil calmness and help normalise sleep patterns	*Liver* Detox and clear system. *Lymphatics* To assist with cleansing and detox of immune system.
Common addictions are drugs (prescription and illegal), smoking, alcohol, food and sex. Causes: • addictive personality • underlying emotional trauma	*Heart* For emotional support. To counteract feelings of guilt, terror or hatred. To promote comfort, confidence and feelings of self-worth	*Kidneys* To remove toxins and increase activity. *Solar plexus* To normalise breathing patterns. To provide

ADDICTION (*cont.*)	Key reflex	Other reflex areas and reason
• physical or mental abuse.		comfort and peace of mind.
Note: A treatment should never be given to a person under the influence of drugs or alcohol		*Self-treatment* Hand reflex points for all of the above to help with sudden cravings and to back up treatments. Also helps clients to take responsibility for their own recovery

ANOREXIA NERVOSA	Key reflex	Other reflex areas and reason
An eating disorder which mainly affects young women – but now men are also increasingly likely to suffer. Characterised by severe weight loss and avoidance of food. Illogical fear of fatness and obesity. Very difficult to treat and can be fatal in extreme cases. Causes:	*Pituitary and all endocrine system* To aid re-balancing of emotional and physical health. *Heart* To help with comfort, confidence and feelings of self-worth.	*Spleen* To assist with energy levels and boost the immune system. *Brain and Spine* To balance and support the nervous system. *Solar Plexus* To assist with supporting the abdominal organs. To help calm, balance and relax. To combat self-
• psychological disorder	*Head and Neck* To help combat tightness, stress and congestion.	

ANOREXIA NERVOSA (*cont.*)	Key reflex	Other reflex areas and reason
• distorted image of body • not fully known or understood.	Note: Bulimia is eating to excess followed by self-induced vomiting. Treat all areas as above but with extra work to digestive and head reflexes.	hatred and obsessional habits.

ARTHRITIS	Key reflex	Other reflex areas and reason
Inflammation of a joint or joints. Can vary from mild ache and stiffness to severe pain and joint deformity. There are many forms of arthritis: osteoarthritis, rheumatoid arthritis, Stills disease (juvenile arthritis), infective arthritis and seronegative arthritis. Causes: • ageing process • obesity • extreme wear and tear • genetic.	Note: For treatment of osteoarthritis only. *Adrenals* To aid production and secretion of cortisone to reduce joint inflammation and pain. *Reflexes of affected joints* To help affected area by stimulating circulation and nerve supply to joint. *Parathyroids* To help with balance of calcium and potassium levels and muscle tension	*Kidneys* To assist with waste product removal around joints. *All spinal reflexes* To increase flexibility and nerve supply, especially: 5c/6c neck 7c shoulder/elbow 1t lower arm, wrist and hand 9t adrenals 1 to 5L for lower back, upper and lower legs and feet. (see Figure 15) *Liver* To assist with filtration of toxins.

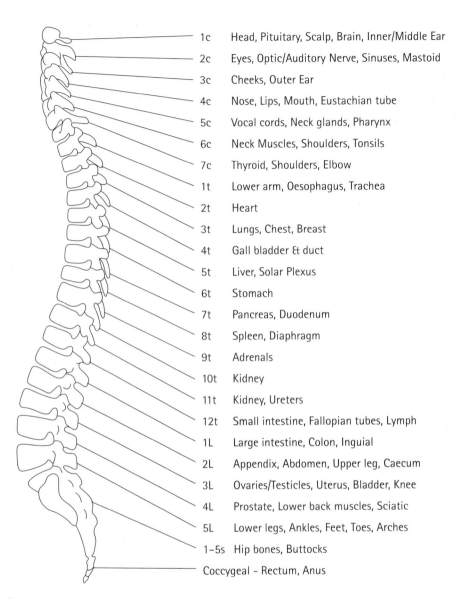

1c	Head, Pituitary, Scalp, Brain, Inner/Middle Ear
2c	Eyes, Optic/Auditory Nerve, Sinuses, Mastoid
3c	Cheeks, Outer Ear
4c	Nose, Lips, Mouth, Eustachian tube
5c	Vocal cords, Neck glands, Pharynx
6c	Neck Muscles, Shoulders, Tonsils
7c	Thyroid, Shoulders, Elbow
1t	Lower arm, Oesophagus, Trachea
2t	Heart
3t	Lungs, Chest, Breast
4t	Gall bladder & duct
5t	Liver, Solar Plexus
6t	Stomach
7t	Pancreas, Duodenum
8t	Spleen, Diaphragm
9t	Adrenals
10t	Kidney
11t	Kidney, Ureters
12t	Small intestine, Fallopian tubes, Lymph
1L	Large intestine, Colon, Inguial
2L	Appendix, Abdomen, Upper leg, Caecum
3L	Ovaries/Testicles, Uterus, Bladder, Knee
4L	Prostate, Lower back muscles, Sciatic
5L	Lower legs, Ankles, Feet, Toes, Arches
1–5s	Hip bones, Buttocks
Coccygeal -	Rectum, Anus

Figure 15 Spinal reflexes

ASTHMA	Key reflex	Other reflex areas and reason
Recurrent attacks of breathlessness accompanied by wheezing and coughing	*Lungs* To relieve congestion and aid regulated breathing.	*Chest* For relaxation of chest muscles.
or Narrowing of bronchioles and spasm of involuntary tissue of bronchi causing difficulty in exhalation.	*Bronchi* To relax and increase blood flow to area	*Solar plexus* For stress release. To help with panic reaction.
Causes:		*Diaphragm* For stress release/to aid breathing.
• Allergy e.g. house dust mite; some drugs; tobacco smoke; food additives, etc.		*Pituitary* To stimulate hormone production.
• Pollution • Viral • Bacterial • Stress/Anxiety		*Adrenals* To aid production of hydrocortisone/ corticosteroids/reduce inflammation/combat allergic response.
		Lymphatics To encourage removal of bacteria/toxins and stimulate immune system.
		Hypothalamus To normalise response of sympathetic nervous system.

BACK PAIN/HIP PAIN/ SACRO ILIAC PAIN	Key reflex	Other reflex areas and reason
Pain in the muscles, joints and ligaments causing muscular spasms and restricted movements. It could effect the thoracic, lumbar, sacral, coccyx or sacro iliac and hip areas. In most cases pain affects soft tissue and in extreme cases prolapsed discs can occur. Causes: • poor posture • standing or sitting for long periods of time • sport or impact injuries • lifting, over exertion • pregnancy • wrong mattress.	*All spinal-cervical/ thoracic/lumbar/sacral/ coccyx* Also include work across the spine to treat nervous system. To help with spinal flexibility, relaxing of muscles and relieving strain. *All sciatic* If pain is in lower back or if nerves are affected. Calms and relaxes area.	*Solar plexus* To relieve tension and tightness and to calm breathing patterns. *Chronic lower back helper areas* To reinforce key reflexes. *Adrenals* For anti-inflammatory effect. *Knee/hip/lower back* To reinforce key reflexes if pain is affecting these areas. *Sacro iliac link point* To balance and stabilise the areas. *Shoulder* To ease pain and relax area if upper thoracic is affected.

BEREAVEMENT	Key reflex	Other reflex areas and reason
Loss of a loved one i.e. wife, husband, child, partner, friend etc.	*Heart reflex* To release grief and help with the healing process. Comfort towards feelings of despair and sadness.	*Diaphragm* To assist in release of tightness in chest and help normalise breathing and sleeping patterns.
	Pituitary To balance emotional health.	*Endocrine* For emotional health.
		Spine and Brain To help balance the nervous system.
		Pineal To regulate sleep pattern.
		Opening and Closing movements Extra attention in order to provide comfort.

CHRONIC FATIGUE	Key reflex	Other reflex areas and reason
Extreme tiredness all the time. Muscles ache and feel heavy. Lack of energy. Rest does not improve feelings of lethargy. Difficulty concentrating.	*Pituitary* To balance the endocrine system and achieve hormonal stability.	*All endocrine glands* To balance hormonal system. *Pineal/Hypothalamus* To help regulate

CHRONIC FATIGUE (cont.)	Key reflex	Other reflex areas and reason
Causes: • stress • post viral • emotional trauma.	*Thymus* To stimulate the immune system.	autonomic responses. To aid biorhythms.
	Spleen To increase energy and boost immune system.	*Spine* To balance central nervous system.
		Diaphragm/Solar plexus To relax entire abdominal area and improve blood supply.
		All lymphatic To balance and boost immune system and stimulate lymphatic drainage.
		Brain To help neurological function.
		Liver To help with energy levels and nutrients.
		Cardiac/Heart To assist with circulation.

| --- | --- | --- |
| Can manifest with several of the following symptoms: sinus congestion, sneezing and coughing, muscular aches and pains, runny nose and eyes, sore throat.

Causes:
• infection caused by a variety of viruses. | Note: Do not treat if client has a very high temperature.

Sinuses
To aid relief of congestion. To assist in mucus drainage and to relieve pain.

Thymus
To help boost the immune system to fight infection.

Head and Neck
To help combat tightness, stress and congestion. | *Lymphatics*
To assist with fighting infection and removal of toxins.

Lungs
To help combat congestion, tightness and coughing.

Ears and Eustachian tube
To assist with clearing congestion and relieving pain. |

CONSTIPATION	Key reflex	Other reflex areas and reason
Difficulty in passing stool. Dry painful sluggish bowel movements. Causes: • poor diet, not enough fibre, fruit and vegetables etc.	*Colon* To assist with the breakdown and removal of waste. *Small Intestine* To stimulate and aid the	*Pancreas* To help with the secretion of digestivejuices. *Stomach* To help with the breaking down of foods.

CONSTIPATION (*cont.*)	Key reflex	Other reflex areas and reason
• dehydration – lack of water balance • stress.	contracting of the intestine, to help removal of waste.	*Solar plexus* To help normalise metabolic function of the abdominal organs.
	Liver/Gall bladder To secrete bile which has a mild laxative effect and aids better digestion.	

CRAMP	Key reflex	Other reflex areas and reason
Involuntary contraction and tightening of muscles. Causes: • restricted circulation • poor diet • fatigue.	*Thyroid/Parathyroid* To help regulate muscle tension. *Knee/Hip/Lower back* To help normalise blood circulation to entire body and to relax muscles.	*Cardiac/Lungs* To assist with oxygen levels. *Lymphatics* To aid removal of waste products and toxins.

CYSTITIS	Key reflex	Other reflex areas and reason
Inflammation of the inner lining of the bladder leading to frequent desire to pass urine, incomplete voiding of urine, burning or stinging pain and sometimes foul-smelling urine.	*Bladder* To improve blood supply to area, relax and help normalise function. *Kidneys and Ureter* To ensure optimum functioning	*Vagina and urethra* To calm and normalise associated area. *Adrenals* To help combat inflammation.

CYSTITIS (*cont.*)	Key reflex	Other reflex areas and reason
Causes: • bacterial infection • poor personal hygiene • bladder stone • enlarged prostate gland • bladder tumour • congenital constriction or introduction of catheter • abnormality of urethra • diabetes predisposes • trauma to urethra from sexual activity • emotional stress.	throughout the rest of the system.	*Lower lymphatics* To help combat infection and assist with removal of debris. *Lumbar spine* To balance nerve supply to area.

DEPRESSION	Key reflex	Other reflex areas and reason
Feelings of sadness, hopelessness and a sense of reduced emotional well-being. Loss of interest in life. Can lead to anxiety attacks, fear etc. Causes: • traumatic life event (death, accident etc.)	Note: **Always treat as near to onset as possible.** *Pituitary* To aid balance of hormonal system. *Thyroid and Parathyroid* To help combat muscle tension.	*Lungs* To assist with oxygen levels. *Heart Reflex* To help combat feelings of fear and hopelessness and to ease the emotional trauma.

DEPRESSION	Key reflex	Other reflex areas and reason
• can occur for no apparent cause • extreme physiological stress.	*Solar plexus* To help combat tightness and stress. To help calm and normalise breathing.	*Spinal reflexes* To assist with balance of nervous system. *Spleen* To provide energy and combat exhaustion. *Adrenals* To assist normalisation and balance and combat stress.

DIVERTICULITIS	Key reflex	Other reflex areas and reason
Small protruding sacs in the wall of the intestine (or colon). Diverticulitis is inflammation of the diverticula in the intestine often caused by perforation or rupture of diverticula. This condition can lead to narrowing of the intestine wall.	*Colon* To help normal function and improve blood supply to area. *Small intestine* To normalise function and stimulate regular bowel movement.	*Adrenals* Production of hydrocortisone. To reduce tissue inflammation. *Lumbar spine* For nerve function to area. *Chronic Achilles area* Helper area to colon. *Lower lymphatics* Encourage drainage/

DIVERTICULITIS (cont.)	Key reflex	Other reflex areas and reason
		removal of waste and toxins.
		Rectum To ease passage of waste.
		Spleen For possible blood loss/to stimulate immune system.
		Solar plexus/Diaphragm General relaxation and autonomic nerve supply.
		Entire digestive tract To relax and normalise function and stimulate peristaltic action.

Task 46 • a) What are diverticula?
b) What is diverticulitis?
c) Name the key reflex area and two other areas that could be given particular attention to help ease the complaint, and give a reason for each.

Task 47 • A client who suffers from asthma comes for treatment:
a) i) Describe this condition.
   ii) Give two possible causes or triggers.
b) Name the key reflex area and two other areas that could be given particular attention to help ease the complaint, and give a reason for each.

Task 48 • A client suffering from cystitis comes for treatment.
   a) i) Describe this condition.
      ii) Give two possible causes or triggers.
   b) Name the key reflex area and two other areas that could be given particular attention to help ease the complaint, and give a reason for each.

ECZEMA/ CONTACT DERMATITIS	Key reflex	Other reflex areas and reason
The skin is the largest organ of elimination. Eczema or contact dermatitis can affect the skin in local areas and cause local inflammation, redness, itching, weeping and blistering.	*Lymphatics* To boost immunity. To regulate removal of toxins. To stimulate healing.	*Spinal reflexes* To aid function of central nervous system, thus balancing function of eliminatory organs.
Causes:	*Liver* To detoxify.	*Endocrine System including adrenals* To regulate hormonal function and stimulate anti-inflammatory response.
• stress • allergy (diet, environmental) • hereditary • fabrics, detergents • metals.	*Kidneys* To stimulate renal process and aid elimination.	

FUNGAL INFECTIONS	Key reflex	Other reflex areas and reason
Many possible manifestations such as: Athlete's foot, candida (imbalance in the gut), skin infections	*Thymus* To stimulate the immune system and help the body fight infection.	*Stomach and intestines* To help balance out good bacteria and cleanse the digestive system.

FUNGAL INFECTIONS (cont.)	Key reflex	Other reflex areas and reason
and nail-bed infections.	*All lymphatics* To help cleanse and detox the system. To assist in the removal of waste products.	*Adrenals* For anti-inflammatory and pain relief. To help with itching. Note: In the case of athlete's foot, if the toe is too infected to treat then use the hand reflexes instead.

GRINDING TEETH	Key reflex	Other reflex areas and reason
Grinding of the teeth, also known as Bruxism. Often occurs at night while sleeping. Can also cause jaw problems and bite may become out of balance. Aching in surrounding tissue. 　Causes: • stress • possible dental problems • unknown factors.	*Solar plexus* To relax and balance in order to assist with more restful sleep. *Pineal* To regulate sleep patterns. *Jaw reflex – upper and lower* To help with inflammation of soft tissue and help restore normal movement.	*All cervical vertebrae* Especially: 3c for teeth and cheeks 4c for mouth 6c for neck muscles, which can often become tight through restless sleep. (See Figure 15) *Self-help* Show client solar plexus and heart reflexes on hands to release worry and tension.

HIATUS HERNIA	Key reflex	Other reflex areas and reason
A protrusion of the upper part of the stomach into the chest through a gap in the diaphragm through which the oesophagus passes; sometimes accompanied by acid reflux and heartburn.	*Diaphragm* To tone, strengthen and normalise function.	*Thoracic spine* To balance nerve impulses to area.
	Stomach To lessen trauma and normalise function.	*Adrenals* To combat inflammation and strengthen muscles.
Causes: • congenital weakness of the diaphragm muscle	*Oesophagus* To relax and normalise function.	*Small intestine* To improve general digestive function.
• unusual pressure from pregnancy • unusual pressure from obesity • smoking • poor posture • lack of exercise (leading to poor muscle tone).		*Solar plexus* To relax entire abdominal area and improve blood supply.

INSOMNIA	Key reflex	Other reflex areas and reason
Insomnia is a disturbance of the normal sleep pattern. Sufferers may have difficulty in falling	*Brain* To relieve tension and normalise function.	*Pituitary* To help normalise functioning throughout endocrine system.

INSOMNIA (*cont.*)	Key reflex	Other reflex areas and reason
asleep or in staying asleep.	*Hypothalamus* To balance responses of autonomic nervous system and regulate sleep patterns.	*Central nervous system* To calm and regulate the nerve impulses throughout (brain and spine).
Causes:		
• stress or worry		
• anxiety		
• depression		
• panic attacks	*Pineal* To regulate secretion of melatonin and balance circadian biorhythms.	*Adrenals* To assist in rebalancing and calming stress response.
• environmental disturbance (e.g. heat, noise)		
• pain		
• lifestyle factors (too much caffeine; lack of exercise; keeping erratic hours)		*Solar plexus* To rebalance parasympathetic response.
• mental illness		
• withdrawal from drugs or medication.		*Diaphragm* To relax and calm.

IRRITABLE BOWEL SYNDROME	Key reflex	Other reflex areas and reason
A condition of abnormal muscle spasm in the bowel, causing intermittent abdominal pain and fluctuations in bowel habits, e.g. constipation, diarrhoea, or a combination of both.	*Colon* To improve blood supply to area relax and help normalise function.	*Chronic Achilles area* General helper area for colon.
	Small intestine To help normalise peristalsis.	*Lumbar spine* To normalise nerve impulses to the area.

IRRITABLE BOWEL SYNDROME (*cont.*)	Key reflex	Other reflex areas and reason
Usually accompanied by sensations of abdominal bloating or swelling, cramp-like pains, wind, mucous or a sensation of incomplete evacuation of the bowels.	*Solar plexus/Diaphragm* To relax abdominal area and help relieve feelings of stress and anxiety.	*Adrenals* For possible allergy/ hypersensitivity and to help normalise muscular contractions and calm inflammation.
Causes: • disturbance of involuntary muscle movement in large intestine • hypersensitivity of bowel due to previous condition such as food poisoning or dysentery • allergy to certain foods • possible disorder in nerves supplying bowels • stress and anxiety.		*Liver/Gall bladder* To normalise flow of bile and lubricate intestines *Digestive tract* To optimise functioning in associated area. *Thyroid/Parathyroid* To regulate the balance of calcium, which is involved in the contraction of muscles. *Hypothalamus* To normalise autonomic responses. *Kidneys* To encourage removal of any toxins.

IRRITABLE BOWEL SYNDROME (*cont.*)	Key reflex	Other reflex areas and reason
		Anal reflex To relax, normalise and ease release of waste.

MIGRAINE	Key reflex	Other reflex areas and reason
A severe, persistent headache, accompanied by disturbances of vision and/or nausea and vomiting.	*Head or Brain* To relax area to improve circulation and normalise function.	*Neck* To improve circulation to release tensions.
Causes:	*Cervical reflexes* To release tension and balance nerve impulses.	*Liver* To encourage detoxification.
• hereditary factors/ genetic predisposition		
• stress/driving oneself to fulfil unrealistic goals		*Kidneys* To encourage detoxification.
• food sensitivity		
• bright or strobing lights		*Adrenals* To aid with any inflammatory reaction, allergic reaction or stress.
• contraceptive pill		
• hormonal		
• trauma		

MIGRAINE (*cont.*)	Key reflex	Other reflex areas and reason
• postural stresses (especially in neck).		*Stomach/Digestive system* To relax and relieve digestive disturbances during an attack.
		Eyes To relieve disturbances and normalise function during an attack.
		Pituitary For emotional and hormonal balance.
		Solar plexus To assist relaxation of abdomen areas and lower anxiety levels.

SINUSITIS	Key reflex	Other reflex areas and reason
Inflammation of the membrane which lines the air-filled cavities around the nose. Sinusitis involves facial pain due to inflammation of the facial sinuses.	*Sinuses* To relax, improve blood supply, relieve congestion, fight infection and clear inflammation of mucous membranes.	*Cervical spine* To stimulate nerve function to area. *Adrenals* To combat inflammation.

SINUSITIS (*cont.*)	Key reflex	Other reflex areas and reason
Causes: • bacterial or viral infection • tooth abscess • severe facial injury • jumping into infected water (which is forced into the sinuses) • allergy • deformity of cartilage of nose • blockage of sinus opening by mucus or polyps.	*Eustachian tubes* To help with associated congestion.	*Upper lymphatics* To encourage removal of waste products and to stimulate immune process to combat infection. *Thymus* To stimulate immune processes to combat infection. *Spleen* To stimulate immune processes to combat infection. *Ileo-caecal valve* To help normalise mucus production. *Kidneys* To aid in removal of toxins from the body.

STIFF NECK	Key reflex	Other reflex areas and reason
Restricted movement and/ or pain in cervical joints. Causes: • muscle spasm • whiplash/injury • poor posture • sports injuries.	*Neck* Front and back to ease tension and improve flexibility. Release muscle spasm and tightness. *Cervical vertebrae* To release tension in each cervical vertebrae. To stimulate nerve function.	*Occipital* To release upper neck tension and prevent further tightness at base of skull and prevent headaches. *Chronic Neck* For pain relief. *Adrenals* For release of cortico steroids for anti-inflammatory and pain relief. *All shoulder reflexes* Can be underlying cause of neck stiffness, due to shoulder and lower back posture.

TINNITUS	Key reflex	Other reflex areas and reason
A ringing, buzzing, whistling, hissing or other noise heard in the ear(s) in the absence of noise in the environment.	*Ear* To relax area, increase blood supply to area and normalise function.	*Deep inner ear/balance point* To relax area, increase blood supply to area and normalise function.

TINNITUS (*cont.*)	Key reflex	Other reflex areas and reason
Causes:	*Cervical reflexes*	*Neck*
• continuous exposure to loud noise	To release tension and balance nerve impulses to area.	To release tension and improve circulation.
• ear disorder, Menieres disease, labyrinthitis, otitis media, etc.		*Head/brain* To improve circulation to area and normalise function.
• blockage of outer ear cana		
• aneurysm of blood vessel in head		*Eustachian tube* To relieve any associated congestion.
• tumour		
• reaction to certain drugs		*Liver* To assist in detoxification.
• head injury		
• emotional response/ stress.		*Kidneys* To assist in detoxification.
		Lymphatics of head and neck To help drain congestion from head and ears.

TINNITUS (*cont.*)	Key reflex	Other reflex areas and reason
		Solar plexus To assist relaxation of abdomen areas and lower anxiety levels.

VARICOSE VEINS	Key reflex	Other reflex areas and reason
Swollen/distended veins just below the surface of the skin, usually in the legs. Blue in appearance. Some people have no symptoms; others have pain, aching and cramps in the affected area. In extreme cases varicose eczema and ulcers can develop. Skin must be kept well moisturised to prevent this occurring.	*Cardiac/Heart reflex* To stimulate the blood circulation. *Hip/Upper Leg/Lower Leg* To stimulate blood flow and reduce swelling/heaviness.	*Lymphatics to groin and legs* To assist in clearance of fluid retention or lymph pooling/swelling. General detox of immune system. *Liver* To cleanse and detox.
Can be present in the rectum as haemorrhoids (piles) or in the testes as varacocile.	**Note:** Never work directly over an area affected by a varicose vein.	*Lumbar vertebrae* To help with blood flow to lower legs.
Elevate when treating. Causes: • the vein walls lose their elasticity and the valve becomes weak,		*Colon/Small intestine* To combat constipation, if present.

VARICOSE VEINS (*cont.*)	Key reflex	Other reflex areas and reason
preventing normal blood flow		
• standing or sitting in the same position for long periods of time		
• constriction of the area		
• hereditary.		

Task 49 • A client suffering from insomnia comes for treatment.
- a) i) Describe this condition.
  - ii) Give two possible causes or triggers.
- b) Name the key reflex area and two other areas that could be given particular attention to help ease the complaint, and give a reason for each.

Task 50 • A client who suffers from sinusitis comes for treatment:
- a) i) Describe this condition.
  - ii) Give two possible causes or triggers.
- b) Name the key reflex area and two other areas that could be given particular attention to help ease the complaint, and give a reason for each.

Task 51 • A client suffering from tinnitus comes for treatment.
- a) i) Describe this condition.
  - ii) Give two possible causes or triggers.
- b) Name the key reflex area and two other areas that could be given particular attention to help ease the complaint, and give a reason for each.

CHAPTER 17

Integrated biology – a brief word

WHAT IS IT?

Integrated biology is a term sometimes used to try to bring together a general understanding of anatomy and physiology with how it affects our behaviour as individuals. For example it is not only important to know that the organs of elimination in the body are the skin, kidneys, liver and lungs but what effect their malfunction would have on the individual, such as tiredness, skin eruptions, bad breath etc.

Another example would be to know that the 'fight or flight' response is the body's response to sudden threat or danger caused by the chemical messages sent from the pituitary and adrenals. The effect on the body would be to raise the heart and pulse rate and make more energy available to the muscles in order to 'fight' the threat or run away from it (flight).

There are many excellent anatomy and physiology books available which will give the underpinning knowledge of the how the body works. An anatomy and physiology book should always from part of your studies, but always try to connect this knowledge with how bodily functions affect the individual.

The next chapters take forward the concept of the body as a whole 'integrated' organism.

CHAPTER 18

Lifestyle

STRESS AND ILLNESS

Each of us carries the potential to contract disease at any time. However, some people become ill while others stay healthy. It is the mental and physical condition of the body that causes subtle changes in hormonal and defence mechanisms, thereby allowing the disease or virus to manifest. By treating the whole person with the 'holistic approach' we enable an equilibrium or homeostasis to be restored where circulation can flow unimpeded and supply nutrients and oxygen to the cells. The body's organs (which are no more than a collection of cells) may then also return to a normal state of function.

It is generally accepted that 75 per cent of all disease is caused by stress. The lifestyle of Western man is the main cause of stress. A certain amount of stress is needed for us to function; it is only when this becomes too much that disease can result. Everyone has different tolerance levels, but we can define stress as being a problem when it fits this definition: the body's reaction to events and emotions that feel outside its conscious control or give a feeling of an inability to cope.

Figure 16 demonstrates some common factors that may trigger an unhealthy amount of stress.

The reflexologist should be alert to stress factors in a client and to indications that the client's coping mechanisms are under undue strain. This information will be gathered during the initial consultations, from the treatments process and from interaction with the client during the treatment process.

The greatest benefit a client can receive from reflexology is relaxation and through this the ability to maintain contact with one's own self and combat the emotional and bodily manifestations of stress in modern-day life. A number of reflex points can greatly assist the body in combating the negative effects of stress:

Reflex Area	Reason
Solar plexus	Aids breathing and relaxation
Diaphragm	Aids breathing and relaxation
Pituitary	Hormonal balance

Reflex Area	Reason
Lungs	Breathing/oxygen balance
Hypothalamus	Balance between endocrine and nervous system
Central nervous system (brain and spine)	Sends messages to calm and balance the whole system
Heart reflex	To release tightness in chest. To centre/ground the client. To release negative emotions.

The pace of life. Quick, too immediate, too pressured.

Attention is directed outwards. We do not accept our sensations and feelings as human beings.

Inability to relax and calm oneself.

Dramatic personal life events or changes (death, birth, moving house, marriage, divorce).

Large amounts of our energy and attention are directed at our head and hands with the demands to do, see and hear more.

The constant threat of violence, murder and other atrocities.

The complex rules and traditions of modern society prevent spontaneous reactions to fear and create feelings of anxiety and tension.

Eating patterns and food intake. The times we eat are often erratic and the food consumed often highly refined or high in additives resulting in the accumulation of toxins which the body finds difficult to dissolve and cleanse from our systems.

The feet and lower parts of the body are neglected through sedentary occupations and transport to and from work.

Natural processes of eliminating the body's waste are suppressed. People often refrain from releasing the body's waste for many hours until social and environmental conditions allow it.

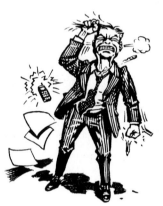

Figure 16

Task 52 • a) Give a one or two sentence general definition of 'stress'.
b) List four factors that may cause or contribute towards stress.
c) List what you consider to be two of the most important reflex areas to treat stress. Give your reason in each case.

ENVIRONMENTAL FACTORS

Environmental factors can also lead to the manifestation of disease. For example a client may report a condition that does not appear linked with a specific medical explanation. In these cases the reflexology practitioner should consider the client's lifestyle and environmental factors. For example if a client has persistent headaches, consider the following environmental factors as contributors:

Environmental factor	Effect on the body that may lead to a headache
Poor posture	Tension in neck muscles, nerve restriction
Poor diet	Lack of adequate nutrients leads to fatigue, inability of body to respond to disease
Irregular eating habits	Low blood sugar levels
Dehydration	Insufficient fluid for kidneys to perform elimination processes satisfactorily
Fluorescent lights	Brightness and flickering can lead to eye strain
Constant loud noise	Leads to pressure on nerves
Excessive computer use	Screen may cause eye strain if used to excess. Link with poor posture

DISEASE AND LIFESTYLE – FINDING THE RIGHT PIL

Another useful tool for the reflexologist in formulating a treatment pattern can be expressed as:

Disease =

Possible

Influencing

Lifestyle

In other words the practitioner should give thought to finding the P.I.L. that can cause, trigger or predispose an individual to a particular condition. Some examples of this theory are:

Disease/condition	Possible Influencing Lifestyle factor (PIL)
Anorexia/Bulimia	Distorted body image
	Low self-worth
	Peer pressure
Arteriosclerosis (heart disease)	Smoking
	High fat/cholesterol diet
	High sugar intake
	Obesity
	Physical inactivity
Arthritis	Dietary factors
	Over use of joints
	Obesity
Asthma	Stress/fear
	Pollution
	Smoking
	Allergies
	Diet
Back pain	Poor posture (standing, sitting etc.)
	Over-exertion
	Occupation (lifting etc.)
	Lack of exercise
Cervical cancer	Many sexual partners
	Early onset of sexual activity
	Stress or trauma
	Smoking
Constipation	Dietary
	Insufficient water
	Irregular eating habits
	Iron supplementation
Depression	Grief (loss of loved one etc.)
	Unemployment/redundancy

Disease/condition	Possible Influencing Lifestyle factor (PIL)
	Relationship problems
	Low self-worth
	Stress/overwork
Diabetes mellitus	Obesity
	Diet high in refined sugars
	Diet low in fibre/unrefined carbohydrates
Eczema/dermatitis	Washing powders
	Dietary
	Cosmetics
	Stress
	Occupational factors (exposure to irritants etc.)
Indigestion	Irregular eating habits
	Rushed meals
	Eating too fast/not chewing
	Too much alcohol with meals
	Eating too frequently
Insomnia	Stress
	Too much caffeine
	Noise pollution
	Eating too late
	Grief/bereavement etc.
Varicose veins	Occupational (standing/sitting)
	Lack of exercise
	Dietary
	Tight clothing

Task 53 • **a)** Name two lifestyle factors that could cause, trigger or predispose someone to each of the following conditions:

     i) Arteriosclerosis
    ii) Diabetes mellitus
   iii) Cervical cancer
   iv) Depression
    v) Varicose veins.

Reflexology: A Complete Guide

b) A client presents with persistent headaches. The doctor finds nothing medically wrong. Give five possible environmental or lifestyle factors that may be contributing to the condition, and give a brief reason for each.

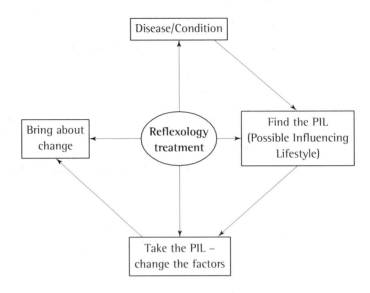

Figure 17

TAKING THE PIL

Once the PIL has been found, it can then be taken by the client as part of the treatment process (as well as the reflexology treatment itself). Taking the PIL together with the treatment may help the effectiveness of the treatment and help with an improvement in some presenting conditions, for example:

Disease/condition	Taking the PIL (effecting a change to lifestyle)
Asthma	Stop smoking
	Avoid walking routes with highly polluted roads
	Take relaxation classes to reduce stress levels
Back pain	Learn to lift heavy items correctly
	Get advice for correct walking posture
	Strengthen the abdominal muscles
	Take a back pain class

Disease/condition	Taking the PIL (effecting a change to lifestyle)
Cystitis	Drink more water
	Take care with personal hygiene
Depression	Talk to someone
	Consider counselling
	Consider joint counselling if in a relationship
	Look for a new interest
	Join a self-help group
	Think about possible causes, e.g. stress at work etc.
Eczema/dermatitis	Wear gloves when cleaning
	Change cosmetics/shower gel to hypoallergenic brands
	Seek advice on diet
	Lower stress levels
	Avoid scratching irritated areas
Insomnia	Develop a bedtime routine
	Play relaxation tapes
	Avoid stimulating activity just before bedtime
	Avoid eating heavy meal just before sleep. Eat two to three hours before bedtime
	Exercise during the day
Varicose veins	Wear support tights or socks
	Improve diet/water intake
	Use stairs rather than lifts or escalators (to improve circulation)
	Wear loose-fitting clothes around the waist

Task 54 • a) What lifestyle advice could you give to someone suffering from insomnia? Give four suggestions.

b) Give two lifestyle suggestions you might recommend to a client to help with cystitis.

AN EXAMPLE OF THE PIL APPROACH

In order to demonstrate the PIL approach, take a client with high blood pressure – also known as hypertension.

Disease/ Condition	Identifying the PIL	Taking the PIL	Reflex areas
Hypertension is blood pressure that is higher than average. High blood pressure occurs because of an increased resistance to blood flow in the blood vessels.	Smoking	• Cutting down on amount consumed • Support groups • Patches etc • Exercise	Lungs Brain Adrenals Lymphatics Endocrine
	Obesity	• Reducing food intake/diet • Exercise • Consult nutritionist	Brain Lymphatics Digestive Endocrine
	Pregnancy	• Breathing exercises • Rest • Gentle exercise	Lighter pressure on Reproductive Endocrine
	Excess alcohol	• Cutting down on amount consumed • Support groups	Liver Kidneys Endocrine Lymphatics
	Sedentary lifestyle	• Exercise	Adrenals Lungs Liver Kidneys

Disease/ Condition	Identifying the PIL	Taking the PIL	Reflex areas
	High salt intake	• Modify diet	Lymphatics
		• Exercise	Vascular system

It is worth noting that exercise is a good PIL against a wide range of factors connected with high blood pressure. This is because it helps to maintain efficient circulation and prevents the deterioration of blood vessels. Other benefits of regular exercise are:

Strengthens the heart and other body muscles

• Maintains joint flexibility

• Improves the efficiency of the respiratory system

• Promotes mental and emotional relaxation

• Uses calories and therefore can help to prevent obesity.

The nature of the exercise depends on the presenting conditions of the individual. It could range from a gentle walk each day to regular workouts at the gym. Be aware that as a reflexologist you are not qualified to give detailed advice on health and fitness activities. If you feel a client requires detailed advice, or has a condition that may require special exercise regimes, advise them to visit their doctor and/or a health and fitness specialist.

Task 55 • a) Define hypertension in one or two sentences.
b) Name four lifestyle factors that may alter normal blood pressure.
c) Give four reasons why exercise is important for good health.

CHAPTER 19

The holistic approach

Reflexology is a form of holistic healing. The term 'holistic' is taken from the Greek word *HOLOS* meaning whole. The holistic approach therefore involves seeing the body as an integrated organism of many parts each of which must function correctly if the others are to do their job.

Three aspects must be involved in order to achieve a feeling of well-being:

- Mind

- Body

- Spirit

As these are viewed as a whole, an imbalance in one will affect the others.

The holistic approach to the reflexology treatment has already been demonstrated throughout the previous chapters, in particular Chapters 11, 12 and 13 and in the PIL approach in Chapter 18. It is the underlying belief that a client's symptoms cannot be treated in isolation, that the whole mind, body, spirit must be taken into account.

For example:

Mind	The repression of emotions, such as anger or grief can
Body	involve a physical increase in bodily tension. The bodily tension is then shown as chronic muscle tension, which is a primary cause of headaches, back pain and poor posture which
Spirit	can then lead to feelings of depression and helplessness.

The holistic approach encourages the client to accept responsibility for their own conditions and to direct their energies and willpower to participate in the healing process. The more the individual is conscious of themselves, their own feelings and perceptions, the more successful the treatment will be. As practitioners we do not cure a person or condition, we assist in the healing process enabling the restoration of energy circulation through the reflexology treatment and the natural deep relaxation it provides.

DISTINGUISHING FEATURES OF THE HOLISTIC APPROACH

- The achievement of homeostasis (equilibrium within the body)

- The balance of mind, body and spirit

- The client taking responsibility by participating in the treatment process

- The therapist helps and supports the client but does not control

- The recognition of external influences and their effect

- The recognition that we are not healing the symptoms alone

- The recognition of the uniqueness of the individual

It becomes obvious, therefore, that the holistic approach demands that each reflexology treatment is given to all points and areas even if the client has no symptoms concerning these areas.

Many other therapies also treat the client with a holistic viewpoint; some of these were explained in Chapter 15.

Task 56 • **a)** Give an example of how, in your opinion, mental attitude/emotions can affect the physical health of the body.
b) Mention five points that are distinguishing features of the holistic approach to health.

PRACTICAL EXAMPLES OF THINKING HOLISTICALLY:

- A visit to the doctors can result in symptoms of an illness being alleviated, but often the patient does not feel better. From an holistic perspective the drugs given may suppress or mask symptoms thus providing relief but not dealing with the main cause of a problem. It is necessary to restore the underlying balance of the body for it to return to full health.

- It may be necessary to treat the mother of a child who has been brought for treatment as the mother may be tense or anxious with worry and this could be passed subconsciously to the child. By helping the mother to be more relaxed it will also help the child.

- Listening can provide relief to a client by giving them an opportunity to talk about a problem. It gives the opportunity to discuss fears and inner thoughts in a non-judgemental atmosphere and helps the client feel valued. It may also help the practitioner to identify patterns that throw light on the client's state of health.

- Continually taking painkillers for a recurrent headache masks the symptoms without discovering the cause. Headaches may be the body's way of showing us that something we are doing is wrong. We should therefore look at possible causes for the headache emanating from our lifestyle and take action to change the trigger for the headaches. Constantly repressing the symptoms could drive the problem further into the body, where it could manifest as a different disorder. It should also be noted that taking some drugs on a regular basis might put a strain on the organs of elimination (liver, kidneys etc.).

- Owning a pet can release chemicals in the brain that can relieve stress and depression and boost the immune system!

- A positive outlook on life can help shed negative mental patterns. Clients can help themselves change their state of mind by undertaking self-help activities such as: meditation, visualisation, affirmations, starting a new hobby or interest, working towards personal goals or getting involved in activities that make one laugh and have fun!

Note: It is not being suggested that the holistic treatment can replace conventional medical treatment. Under no circumstances should a reflexologist recommend that a patient stop taking prescribed drugs. Only the patient's doctor can give medical advice regarding drugs. The reflexologist must refer the patient to their doctor if complications arise which the reflexologist feels are due to the taking of prescribed drugs.

Task 57 • a) A visit to the doctor can result in symptoms of an illness being alleviated, but often the patient still does not feel better. From a holistic perspective, give one reason why this might be so.
  b) What might be a benefit of treating the mother of a child who has been brought to you for treatment?
  c) Give two ways in which your listening skills could benefit your client.

THE HEALING CRISIS

The healing crisis evolves directly from the holistic philosophy. The body may respond to treatment by a severe, but temporary, worsening of symptoms or the appearance of apparently new acute symptoms. This is usually followed by an improvement in the client's condition and may often be a turning point in their illness. There is no set time limit for a healing crisis – it may occur after only one or two treatments or after many treatments and may last from a few hours to a few weeks. It is important to reassure the client that it is a positive sign indicating that the body is responding to treatment. It is also important for the reflexologist to keep monitoring new and acute symptoms and reactions from the treatment to ensure that a prolonged and extreme negative reaction does not occur as this would indicate the need to cease treatments (see Chapter 8).

Task 58 • a) Briefly explain the concept of the healing crisis.
b) List three self-help activities or methods that might help a client to let go of negative mental patterns and develop a more positive outlook on life.

CHAPTER 20

The subtle body

The subtle body is a description often used to represent what some believe to be an energy force flowing through and/or rippling out from the physical body. It has been likened to an electromagnetic energy field, which cannot be seen with the eye but surrounds the body with the unique energy of an individual. Others prefer to call it a life force and believe that it represents different levels of awareness radiating out from the physical body – types of non-physical or subtle bodies such as divine, spiritual and universal.

This subtle body life force can be received and absorbed through:

- fresh food
- touch
- breathing
- meditation/relaxation

If we accept the existence of the subtle body/energy pathway then it follows that, as well as all the other benefits of reflexology, we could also be affecting the subtle body, due to an exchange between client and practitioner. The following effects could therefore be experienced as a direct result of this energy exchange:

- tingling
- pulsating
- cold/chilling
- A sympathetic experience by the practitioner of a client's symptoms
- Momentary discomfort or pain
- heat
- cool breeze off the feet
- sensation of energy flow
- An intuitive insight on the part of the practitioner

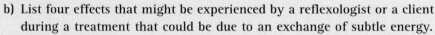

Task 59 • a) Describe what you understand by the subtle body.
b) List four effects that might be experienced by a reflexologist or a client during a treatment that could be due to an exchange of subtle energy.
c) Name two ways in which we receive/absorb the life force or vital energy.

As the subtle body's force flows through and out of the body it is possible that disturbances in the physical body could affect the natural flow of these energies. Mental and physical factors that could effect the subtle bodies are:

- Stress
- Illness
- Pollution
- Pain
- Injury
- Trauma

- Tension
- Fear
- Poor posture
- Lack of exercise
- Emotional rigidity
- Self-absorption

Because the subtle body is 'linked' with the physical body the above factors would influence both the subtle and the physical body. It also follows that a reverse link could be possible, in other words that an imbalance in the subtle body could affect the physical.

The level of energy flow may be affected by the above factors and could be indicated on the feet by:

- dull or no response on reflexes
- numbness or loss of feeling
- damp/clammy feet

- pale colour
- dry, parched skin
- 'empty' areas

Task 60 • **a)** List four mental or physical factors that could impede the flow of life energies through the body.
b) List four indications that could be present on the feet if a client is low in 'vital' energy.

Many other therapies also believe in the subtle body theory, although it may be known under a variety of names such as 'Chi' or 'Vital energy'. Examples of other therapies that use such a philosophy are:

- Acupuncture
- Applied Kinesiology
- Healing

- Radionics
- Colour therapy
- Reiki

Reflexologists who accept the existence of the subtle bodies believe that by working the reflex points it is possible to influence the subtle body by stimulating the energy and restoring a 'natural flow'. It is not, of course, compulsory that the practitioner believe in the subtle bodies theory as it has already been demonstrated that reflexology works on many other levels of the individual.

Task 61 • **Name four therapies that work with therapies that flow through the body.**

CHAPTER 21

Diet and nutrition

As discussed in Chapter 15 the reflexology practitioner must give advice relating only to the reflexology treatment. It is very important that no advice is given that is beyond the competence of the reflexologist. However, it is important to understand the basic functions of the body, and a diet that keeps the body healthy is vital to help it achieve homeostasis (see Chapter 18). It does not mean the reflexology practitioner is qualified to give nutritional advice.

THE BASICS

The body needs food in order:

- to sustain life

- to produce energy

- to build the body and repair physical damage

- to regulate hormonal processes

- to maintain all body processes

- to replace cells.

The basic nutritional components of a balanced diet are carbohydrates, fats, proteins, minerals and vitamins.

VITAMINS AND MINERALS

A balanced intake of vitamins and minerals is considered essential for the healthy function of the body. For example the minerals that are important for bone growth and repair are calcium, phosphorus and magnesium. Iron is important for the body's haemoglobin levels, as lack of iron can cause anaemia (depleted ability of haemoglobin to store oxygen). Iron is present in meat and liver as well as pulses and green leafy vegetables.

With regard to vitamins, vitamin A helps with normal growth, formation of bones and teeth, healthy skin and hair and resistance to infection. It can be found in eggs, dairy produce and liver. It is also present in foods such as peas, potatoes, spinach, carrots and tomatoes that contain beta-carotene, which can be converted into retinol (vitamin A). Vitamin C is present in much fresh fruit. It is necessary for the immune system to function efficiently and because it can help to protect against infections, cancer and heart disease. Vitamin C also provides a valuable source of fibre.

Fibre is important in the diet because it:

- adds bulk to faeces

- aids passage of water through the intestines

- aids normal bowel function

- prevents constipation

- reduces the incidence of bowel disorders

- holds water.

Task 62 • a) Give four reasons why the body needs food.
b) Name four of the basic nutritional components of a balanced diet.
c) Give two reasons why fibre is important in the diet.
d) List two minerals that are important for bone growth and repair.

Task 63 • a) Give two reasons why the body needs vitamin A.
b) Name two food sources that contain vitamin A.
c) Name two types of food that contain iron.
d) What effect would iron deficiency have on the body?

MODERN FOOD PRODUCTION

Many clients have concerns about the amount of pre-cooked and pre-prepared foods they are eating, and the affect it may have on their health. Some of the main issues concern:

- the use of chemical sprays (fertilizers, herbicides, pesticides)

- the use of hormones in animal husbandry

- intensive farming

- genetic engineering

- lengthy storage times

- chemical ripening processes

- irradiation
- refining natural foods
- chemical additives
- added sugar
- pre-cooked foods
- fast foods
- use of 'unnatural' components in animal feed.

In the same way many clients have concerns about refined foods because they do not contain sufficient quantities of vitamins, minerals and fibre. They may also increase tooth decay, due to added sugars. Preservatives, colourings and added chemicals may also place a strain on the body's digestive processes, leading to constipation or other bowel problems.

While debate still continues over the effect of modern food production methods on the body, the best general advice is to try to eat a balanced diet, which may consist of some of the above, but should also include fresh fruit and vegetables and contain nothing in excess.

FOOD SENSITIVITY

Reflexologists may also observe that certain foods can produce sensitive or allergic reactions, for example wheat, nuts, dairy products, tomatoes, shellfish, caffeine etc. It is also possible that some foods may be linked with certain conditions, so-called food allergies. If you suspect a client is suffering from a food-related allergic condition then a referral to a qualified nutritionist would be appropriate. The reflexology treatment will certainly help the body to combat the allergic effect, but a more detailed investigation into the precise food-related triggers would be beneficial.

The following conditions may be associated with food allergy or sensitivity:

- Asthma
- Eczema
- Rhinitis (runny nose)
- Migraine
- Irritable Bowel Syndrome
- Coeliac disease
- Catarrh
- Sinus problems
- Arthritis
- Depression
- Hyperactivity
- M.E.
- Acne
- Psoriasis
- Irritable bladder.

Task 64 • a) Give three reasons why refined foods are considered bad for health.

b) Give three conditions that may be associated with food allergy or food sensitivity.

c) Name four common foods that may give rise to sensitivity or an allergic reaction in some people.

CHAPTER 22

Presentation, client care and health and hygiene

A professional image is vital to a successful reflexologist. In later chapters there is information regarding marketing and publicity and working as a reflexologist *but* there is no more important issue than that of the presentation of the reflexologist. Within the first 30 seconds of meeting a client their vital initial impressions are formed. This will set the tone for your future relationship with them. Get this wrong and it is very difficult to back track; get it right and they are more likely to return again and again. The advice given here is relevant to reflexology students as well as those beginning or already in practice. A 'practice' represents a global term referring to all reflexologists who treat a client base on a regular basis. The points made are relevant to the practitioner working from home or from treatment rooms.

PRESENTATION

The presentation of a practice is **of vital importance**.

CLEANLINESS

The treatment room should be kept clean and dust-free at all times with adequate ventilation. All couch/pillow covers should be clean and spare sets should be available at all times. New clean towels and couch roll (tissue) should be used for each client. Antiseptic/sterile wipes should be used on the feet before treatment. A bin with a top (pedal bin type) should be available for disposal of used couch roll and other items. These measures are important in order to prevent cross-infection and to promote health and safety.

Toilet and hand-washing facilities should be available. A blanket should be available in case a client feels cold.

DECOR

The style of your room and its contents are, to a certain extent, a matter of personal preference. Some practitioners prefer a semi-clinical approach with light clean colours and furniture while others prefer a warmer, softer atmosphere. There are, however, some basic ground rules that should be observed:

COLOUR

There are many theories as to the most beneficial colours to use in a treatment room. Blue is often thought of as a cool, healing colour while green is said to induce calm and tranquillity. The two colours that should be avoided are white and black. A completely white room is far too bright and clinical. It is completely impersonal and is likely to dazzle clients and cause headaches and tension. The use of white sparingly, for instance on skirting boards and doorframes only, and in eggshell rather than gloss is acceptable. Black is too negative and is likely to engulf the client, causing depression and anxiety. Shades of white or a white background with softer colours superimposed is much better for creating a clean yet gentle atmosphere. Avoid harsh or overwhelming colour combinations (e.g. green with pink and orange, stripy wallpaper with floral borders and violet skirting boards).

DECORATION

Carefully chosen pictures in frames can add a relaxed feel. Avoid clinical diagrams and anatomical charts etc. Always display your professional certificates and qualifications along with insurance documentation and local authority licence. It may be better to display these in a waiting area if one is in use, otherwise in the treatment room itself.

FURNITURE

Try to provide an area away from the treatment couch or chair in which to sit and talk to clients. You may wish to use a desk and chairs or two comfortable arm chairs. This, again, depends on your individual approach.

A cabinet or storage case for client treatment records is essential – this should be lockable in order to maintain confidentiality. This facility could also be used for storing stationery, journals and correspondence. A display shelf is also desirable in order to draw your client's attention to relevant products or interesting books/journals.

A coat hanger should be available along with a suitable place to store client's shoes.

Task 65 • a) **List six important considerations when designing and equipping a treatment room.**
b) **Give two reasons why hygiene in your practice is important.**

SELF PRESENTATION

Once again the practitioner's style of dress and presentation is largely a matter of personal choice but one should always aim to present a clean, professional image.

DRESS

Some practitioners prefer to wear white garments in the form of jogging wear or slacks and shirt while others wear all forms of colour coordinated dress. The presentation of the practitioner forms a very powerful first impression and for this reason you should think very carefully about what you wear. For example:

WHITE COAT

Appearing in a white doctor's coat may present a clean, clinical image but may trigger undesirable hospital/dentist/pain/anxiety association with your client, perhaps undoing any good that you are about to administer!

JEANS AND T-SHIRT

Appearing in jeans and a t-shirt may present too much of a casual look and the client could mistake you for another patient or think it is your day off! They may think that the treatment you are about to administer is going to be along the same lines!

Whatever you decide is an appropriate dress style for your client base and image, it may be worth considering wearing a name badge stating your membership of professional associations as a clear mark of your professionalism.

SELF

Always ensure that your nails are clean and short and that your hands are spotless. Always wash your hands thoroughly after each treatment. Keep your hair well groomed so that it does not continually fall in your face during treatments.

Be careful if you eat spicy foods or are a smoker as these smells can often linger on the breath and clothes for several hours. Therefore they should be avoided due to your close proximity to clients. If you do indulge use a mouthwash before commencing your treatments. Strong aftershaves or perfumes should be avoided for the same reason although deodorants must, of course, be worn.

Task 66 • List what you consider to be four important factors in the way practitioners present themselves. Give your reason in each case.

HEALTH AND SAFETY

Ensure that all electrical equipment has been correctly installed and that plugs have the correct fuses and are not in a damaged or dangerous condition. Make sure that your treatment couch and/or chair is regularly maintained to avoid the possibility of injury due to loose joints or sharp edges.

Always ensure that a first-aid kit is within easy reach for emergencies. Protective plastic gloves should form part of the kit.

Other first-aid measures could include: a sugary drink in case a client suffers a hypoglycaemic attack (diabetic), a paper bag in case of hyperventilation and an eye bath in case irritants enter the eye.

It is strongly recommended that all reflexologists undertake at least a one-day first-aid course so that basic first aid can be given in an emergency situation. The key tasks for a first aider in an emergency situation are to:

- assess the situation
- make the area safe
- assess the casualty(ies)
- give emergency aid
- get help

It is recommended that a reflexologist is able to give emergency resuscitation and understand the recovery position and when to use it. In addition a reflexologist should be confident to deal with the following: a hypoglycaemic attack, hyperventilation, fainting and nosebleeds – although they are not common events during a reflexology treatment!

CHAPTER 23

Keeping records, the ethics of practice and support systems

KEEPING RECORDS – CONFIDENTIALITY

We have already discussed the importance of keeping client consultation and treatment cards confidential. As a reminder, you are in a position of trust and responsibility. For the records to remain confidential you must take the following action:

- Keep them in a secure place, preferably a locked cabinet.

- Do not allow others access to your client records

- Do not discuss personal details of your clients with others. You may, of course, need to discuss details of various clients' conditions with other healthcare professionals or tutors or for research projects. In these cases any of the client's identifying details such as name, address and doctor should be withheld. All other details that do not personally identify the client can then be presented anonymously thus protecting the client's confidentiality.

THE ETHICS OF PRACTICE

A practitioner should always maintain the highest standards of conduct so as to instil confidence in and trust from clients. It is for this reason that all reflexologists should belong to a professional reflexology organisation.

When joining a reflexology organisation the practitioner will be required to agree to a set of rules and regulations regarding their conduct and the practice of reflexology. These rules and regulations are often referred to as a Code of Ethics or a charter of responsibilities towards clients. By belonging to a reflexology organisation the practitioner will have the reassurance and support of an experienced group of fellow reflexologists. The public will be reassured that not only is their reflexologist professionally qualified, but will act with integrity. The public will also feel reassured that there is an established structure that will listen to and act upon genuine complaints.

Below are examples of rules that will typically appear in a code of ethics document:

- Members shall not claim to cure.

- Publicity should be accurate and discreet in accordance with the British Code of Advertising practice.

- Members should treat clients according to their own personal needs and not according to gender, ethnic origin or sexual orientation.

- Members shall not seek to attract business unfairly or unprofessionally or in any way to the discredit of reflexology.

- Members should only practise within the limits of their training and competency.

- Members shall not engage in conduct likely to bring the organisation into disrepute such as: dishonesty, indecency or other criminal offences (this would almost certainly result in disciplinary proceedings being taken against the reflexologist by the membership organisation).

- All information is to be kept confidential.

As a reflexologist you have a duty of care towards your client, but this does not mean that you have to treat all those who request a treatment. There are many valid reasons why a reflexologist may refuse to treat a client. For example:

- You feel unsafe or uncomfortable with them.

- You are too personally involved.

- They have made insulting or derogatory remarks about you to other people.

- They refuse to consult a GP regarding serious symptoms.

- There is a clash of personalities.

- They have refused to pay for previous treatments.

- You are too busy to take on new clients.

- They have offensive smell or appearance.

In the final analysis it is the professional judgement of the reflexologist as to who they treat, provided such judgements are reasonable and not incompatible with any code of ethics.

 Task 67 • a) What are two of the main reasons for establishing a Code of Ethics for reflexologists?
b) Name three types of misconduct, which could result in disciplinary procedure against a member.
c) Give three reasons why you might refuse to treat a client.

SUPPORT NETWORKS

As you begin to treat as a qualified reflexologist you may feel a client is in need of the services of other caring/support organisations. This is a sensitive area and the practitioner must be certain that the information is requested by the client or will be welcomed by them as a continuation of the treatment process.

It will be useful for you to build up a contact list of organisation/support networks, which may be helpful to future clients. Examples of such support networks are:

- Relate
- The Samaritans

- Alcoholics Anonymous
- Age Concern.

There are many more support and self-help groups providing advice on a whole range of topics, for example:

- Bereavement
- Arthritis

- Depression and stress
- Cancer

- Sexual abuse/rape
- AIDS/HIV.

- Asthma

Many of these groups have local contact numbers that you can find from information providers such as the library, Citizens Advice Bureau, Thompson Local/Yellow Pages, the local council and the Internet (reliable sites only!).

Task 68 • a) Why should practitioners be aware of local and national support systems?
b) How might you find out about the existence of organisation and support networks? Give three sources.

CHAPTER 24

Starting out – modes of work and personal safety

MODES OF WORK

As a newly qualified reflexologist there are several decisions you need to make before starting your own practice. They may be long-term aims which, although not realistic at the present time, should be seriously considered in order to give your work direction and motivation.

Ask yourself the following questions . . .

DO YOU WANT TO WORK FULL-TIME OR PART-TIME?

If you decide you want to work full-time you may invest a larger proportion of your savings and/or current earnings into marketing and publicity to increase your client base. You may start by working part-time and gradually build up enough business to reduce the hours of your present occupation with a view to ceasing your current employment altogether.

If you wish to work part-time only you may not need to market yourself as vigorously and may wish to pick and choose your clients or specialise in a particular area. Your hours of work may be more variable if you have another source of income.

DO YOU WANT TO WORK FROM BUSINESS PREMISES, FROM HOME OR TRAVEL TO CLIENTS?

The cost of maintaining and/or hiring a shop or treatment room should be remembered if you want to work from business premises. They may, however, attract passing trade and project a more professional image.

Working from home involves setting aside a room and meeting the required standards of Local Authority Licensing Laws (see Chapter 26). The type of home in which you live (e.g. house, flat, maisonette) and restrictions in the freehold, lease or rental agreement must be considered. Savings over leased business premises can be considerable.

Location of your home, parking, neighbours and tax/community charge requirements are also factors. Vulnerability may be an issue – you could feel uneasy while alone with some people.

Travelling to clients involves transport expenses and carrying equipment. Again, vulnerability must be considered. Premises and licensing costs are, however, eliminated leaving more profit.

DO YOU WANT TO BE SELF-EMPLOYED OR AN EMPLOYEE?

Self-employment requires registration for tax and National Insurance purposes. Income/expenditure accounts must be kept and tax paid on earnings above a certain limit. Insurance for accident or illness must also be considered along with pension/investment plans. Self-employment does, however, allow total flexibility and gives the freedom to pursue new initiatives. Earnings are limited only by your energy and imagination!

Being employed by a third party relieves you from the administrative burdens of self-employment but may limit your flexibility and earnings.

DO YOU WANT TO WORK WITH OTHERS OR ALONE?

Partnerships are an effective way of splitting costs and sharing expertise as well as expanding customer contacts. However, legal contracts and profit agreements must be undertaken to ensure that there are no problems in the future.

Working alone allows total freedom. Isolation can be a problem.

Sharing premises with others, working from a group clinic or forming a cooperative may be a midway solution. It could permit easy referral between practitioners, allow cost sharing and combat isolation. It could, however, also mean that you may not have total control over the surroundings and may have to compromise on hours worked due to room availability.

Figure 18 brings together all the elements into a starting out flow chart.

Task 69 • a) Give three advantages and three disadvantages of running a clinic from home.
b) Give two advantages and two disadvantages of working from a group complementary clinic.

Task 70 • a) Give three advantages and three disadvantages of being self-employed.
b) Give three advantages and three disadvantages of carrying out home visits to clients.

PERSONAL SAFETY

Although working as a reflexologist is a very safe profession it is one that involves working in close personal contact with others whom you may not know well. It is sensible to take precautions when arranging to see clients for the first time.

STARTING OUT – GO WITH THE FLOW

QUESTION ONE

Do you want to work FULL-TIME?

↓

Invest a larger proportion of savings/income in marketing. Decrease other work gradually if possible.

Do you want to work PART-TIME?

↓

Work by recommendation. Bear in mind unsocial hours/other commitments. Strike the right balance.

QUESTION TWO

Do you want to work from home?

↓

Set aside a room.

Get Local Authority Licence (if needed).

Check restrictions in lease/freehold etc.

Consider neighbours/parking tax/insurance issues.

ADVANTAGES: Economical overheads, flexible working.

DISADVANTAGES: Legal restrictions. Available room. Unable to escape. Neighbours. Car parking etc.

Do you want to travel to clients?

↓

Get transport.

Ensure proper business car insurance.

ADVANTAGES: No premises overheads. Licence not required. Flexible working.

DISADVANTAGES: Vulnerability. Carrying of equipment etc.

Do you want to work from business premises?

↓

Lease premises or room.

Check lease/rental contract for conditions/restrictions.

Get Local Authority Licence (if needed).

ADVANTAGES: Attract passing trade. Raise awareness.

DISADVANTAGES: Cost of lease/business rates etc.

QUESTION THREE

Do you want to be self-employed?

↓

Inform tax office of your trade and apply for self-employed status.

Keep accurate income/expenditure accounts.

Consider accident insurance/pension plans etc.

ADVANTAGES: Flexibility of earnings. Ability to persue own initiatives. Able to form partnership/cooperative. Limited Company status may limit personal liability.

DISADVANTAGES: Insecurity. Tax affairs. Extra stress. Personal liability (except LTD. company). Isolation (consider a partnership or cooperative).

Do you want to be an employee?

↓

Seek employment by companies or organisations.

Work according to employers' contract.

ADVANTAGES: No burdens of self-employment.

DISADVANTAGES: Limited opportunities for increase in earnings.

Limited career flexibility.

Figure 18. The starting out flow chart

SAFETY CHECKS

WHEN TAKING A TELEPHONE BOOKING FROM A FIRST-TIME CLIENT:

Question	Reason
Where did you get my number?	Establishes if the client is from recommendation or another source. Recommended clients at least are known by one or more of your current clients.
May I take your home address and home and work telephone numbers, so that I can contact you in case I have a problem with your appointment, or need to drop you a reminder note.	Always get all this information so that you are sure the client is genuine. A genuine client will not withhold these details. Do not just accept a mobile telephone number. Also make sure you ring at least one of the numbers to confirm the appointment so that you can be sure it is genuine. A confirm receipt appointment card sent through the post is also a good idea.
For home visits: Do you live in a house or flat? Is there somewhere for me to park near your home and is the area well lit? Are there any access difficulties?	Establishes the viability of a home visit and the type of access available. Allows you to assess the risk to your safety.

WHEN TREATING THE CLIENT:

Action	Reason
For home visits: Take a mobile phone and a personal alarm. Always tell someone you trust the name, address and telephone	Allows you to stay in control and establishes a safety net in case of problems.

Action	Reason
number of the client you are visiting. Tell them how long you will be and arrange to ring them when you have finished. Tell them to raise the alarm if they have not heard from you by a pre-agreed time.	
Make sure you have a planned exit route. Do not put the client between you and the doorway. Have a personal alarm in the room.	Allows for an escape in an emergency situation.
Arrange for someone to be in the building when you are seeing a client for the first time at a clinic or at your home. If this is not possible then leave a TV or radio on in another room to show signs of other people being around. Book other regular clients before and after a first-time client.	Increases your personal safety. Help is closer to hand.

As previously mentioned, reflexology is a very safe profession, but it is sensible to take basic precautions in the very unlikely event that there is a threat to your personal safety. There is another vital precaution you can take:

Listen to your own intuition – if a person does not look or sound right or a situation looks or feels odd then listen to these subconscious messages. Do not ignore them. You are perfectly entitled not to see a client or to make up an excuse and leave a home visit if you feel uncomfortable. Sometimes it is impossible to describe or quantify this intuitive early warning light but many people describe it as 'Something just didn't feel right' or 'I had a strange feeling about that place'. Where your own personal safety is at risk do not suppress these intuitive feelings – they are there for a purpose!

There are many excellent sources of free advice and guidance for the safety of lone workers, such as the Suzy Lamplugh Trust. Your local library or Citizens Advice Bureau will have further details.

CHAPTER 25

Advertising and marketing

When thinking about publicity bear in mind the following factors:

- Who are your main user groups and how can they be contacted?

- How much money are you prepared to spend?

- How much business do you want to generate?

- What image do you wish to project?

THE BASICS

There are a few basic publicity and marketing items that should form part of every practitioner's business.

BUSINESS CARDS

A traditional form of publicity which instantly presents a professional image and ensures you a place in a prospective client's memory (and filofax).

Business cards can be among the cheapest forms of publicity depending on the type and size chosen. If you are working on a limited budget the quickest and cheapest way to obtain a reasonable starting amount is to use the ready made computerised machines that can be found in some large stationery shops and shopping centres. For a few pounds it produces, within a few minutes, 25 large or 50 small cards from your typed in script. If you prefer to have something more elaborate and can use a PC then there are many software packages that can produce business cards. Print shops could also be approached. These professionally produced cards will cost more but become cheaper for larger orders.

SERVICE LEAFLET

A leaflet that explains the benefits of the treatment offered along with a brief history of your training and experience is excellent for persuading those hesitant 'would be' clients to undergo treatment. Again the nature of the leaflet will vary according to your budget. It is possible to type your own basic leaflet or engage the services of a printer. Alternatively many of the Reflexology Associations provide standard leaflets for members at a reasonable cost.

POSTER/DISPLAY CARD

An A3 or A4 size poster and/or postcard-type banner can be useful to display in health shops and doctors' surgery (if they are willing). An item such as this, if designed well, will stand out from other haphazardly placed business cards and handwritten notices.

Other desirable items are:

- letter-headed stationery
- appointment cards

- invoices and receipt slips
- compliment slips.

IMPORTANT POINTS

Bear in mind the following points when acquiring the basics:

1. *Presentation*. Always aim to produce a professional image. All material should be printed and/or photocopied. Handwritten material, although 'earthy', does not project an image of efficiency and professionalism and will lose more business than it gains.

2. *Consistency*. Decide on a basic design, which may include a logo or a particular print style, and stick to it. This will provide a recognisable image and will enable customer association.

3. *Credibility*. Always include your name, contact number and relevant qualifications on any publicity.

Task 71 • a) In any advertising what do you consider to be the three most important general principles? Give a reason in each case.
   b) List four items of business stationery that you would consider to be important for the running of your business
   c) What, in your opinion, are three of the most useful pieces of information to include on any publicity information?

GENERATING BUSINESS

Each practitioner has their own preferred method of generating business and no one approach can be considered preferential. The suggestions and comments below will enable the reflexologist to consider the marketing methods best suited to their aspirations. The previous points relating to professional presentation should be followed for all the below methods.

WORD OF MOUTH

This is the cheapest and most effective form of publicity. Once you have successfully treated several clients your business should grow from recommendations. Depending on the amount of work you wish to generate and in order to 'find' your first customers to spread the word you may wish to consider some of the below more direct approaches.

POSTER CAMPAIGNS

A cost-effective way of publicising your skills providing you choose your display places carefully.

For instance placing a poster/card in a newsagent's is not likely to attract customers or, if it does, they may be looking for a different type of service. If you were looking for a well-qualified reflexologist would you look in your local shop? It is much more likely that a poster/card in a health shop, chiropodists/podiatrists or gymnasium will provide you with new clients. If your local GP is open to complimentary treatments his/her surgery is a good place to display a poster. Workplace noticeboards are also a good place to advertise your skills.

MAIL SHOTS (DIRECT MAIL)

A general letter explaining your skills to interested parties is another cost-effective form of publicity. It has limited use for the reflexologist wishing to work independently but is an excellent way of introducing yourself to health clubs and group complimentary practices that may wish to employ the services of a reflexologist. Your service leaflet may also be used for mail shots to appropriate potential customers but would not be as effective as material specifically designed for introductory purposes.

PRESS ADVERTS

Placing advertisements in the local press can generate much interest. However, this form of advertising is expensive and can result in many nuisance calls. Always think very carefully about the phrasing of your advert and ensure it is thoroughly professional. It is desirable not to take cold bookings from people responding to your adverts. Take their name, address and telephone number in order to send them further details, after which they may book an appointment. You should call them back before the appointment to confirm details (see Chapter 24 for more personal safety advice). If they seem at all hesitant in giving particulars do not offer to treat them or give out your working address.

If you have funds available for press adverts it is much better to place a small advert for a prolonged period of time rather than use all your available funds for one large advert.

It may be worth considering specialist magazines and journals as an alternative to the local press. Your target audience is more readily identifiable using this method and may bring more effective results for less outlay. For example British Airways publish an in-house magazine for their staff, many of whom have stressful jobs and may find your services of great benefit. Many large department stores also produce their own staff publications whose readership certainly requires attention for stress and exhaustion.

TALKS AND SEMINARS

These are an excellent way to spread the word. Approach local groups and organisations that may wish you to provide a demonstration and/or lecture on the benefits of reflexology (e.g. Women's Institute, retirement groups, etc.). It may also be worth approaching your local doctor's practice many of whom have user groups that meet regularly to listen to talks and demonstrations on health care.

INTERNET

An internet site can be a useful source of publicity and information, and is inexpensive if you are able to compile it and update it yourself. Having a site will not, in most cases, increase your business until you make people aware of the site address. This should be included in all your other forms of publicity as a place to obtain more information. The internet site can then expand on the basic publicity information and create more interest. When compiling a site keep the first page simple and easy to read with links to other pages, and check that download times from a standard modem are acceptable. As with newspaper advertising please remember your personal safety rules when taking first-time bookings from this source.

It should be remembered that in any publicity or marketing material the reflexologist should not make claims to cure or heal specific problems and ailments but should inform the public of the holistic benefits of the treatment. Gimmicks and free offers should be avoided at all costs as this type of aggressive marketing is incompatible with the professional approach to treatment expected of the practitioner. Gift vouchers and a discount for a course of treatments (paid in advance) are acceptable marketing techniques.

Task 72 • a) Give one advantage and one disadvantage of newspaper advertising.
b) Apart from the above, give four other marketing methods for promoting yourself as a reflexologist.

CHAPTER 26

Legal requirements

Important note:

This chapter relates to England and Wales only. Other countries, regions and states may have different legislation. Contact the relevant authorities or reflexology organisations in the country or region where you live, if outside England and Wales.

In comparison to some other countries, practitioners in the UK enjoy a large amount of freedom to practise complementary therapies, largely due to lack of specific legislation to prevent it. In some other countries it is forbidden to practise certain therapies without first undertaking detailed training to the equivalent of nursing, or in some other countries without first being a doctor.

The lack of specific legislation is largely a combination of historical accident, government inactivity and a lack of a cohesive voice from the various complementary therapy associations and groups. It does not, however, excuse the professional practitioner from adhering to the highest standards of practice, indeed it makes it even more necessary, so that the public can be confident of high standards through self-regulation. This situation may of course change depending on European legislation and government changing attitudes towards regulation in the complementary therapy fields.

For the time being it is important to understand the basics about the law as it affects reflexologists.

The law of England is divided into two main categories: criminal law and civil law.

CRIMINAL LAW

This is contained in Acts of Parliament and governs the conduct of members of the community through the state. These Acts of Parliament are the main areas of the law that concern the reflexologist.

CIVIL LAW

Here, decisions are taken by a court in cases that have come before them. Civil law governs the rights and liabilities of members of the community in relation to one another. This mainly concerns the reflexologist in terms of being sued for professional negligence (see page 205).

Many of the laws detailed below are not explicitly for reflexology practitioners or complementary health practitioners, but were passed by parliament to cover a number of concerns – many of which are, in this day and age, not as relevant as they once may have been. It is, however, important to know the general legislation that could be relevant to reflexology practitioners.

MEDICAL AID AND CHILDREN

No complementary therapy is approved as medical aid under the law. It is against the law for a parent or guardian not to seek medical aid for a child (under 16) who needs it. If a parent or guardian refuses to seek medical aid for a child who needs it the practitioner should obtain a signed statement from the parent or guardian:

I have been warned by_____that according to the law I should consult a doctor concerning the health of my child.

_____Name of child. Signed_____parent or guardian

Signed by witness_____.

Relevance to reflexologists

It is highly unlikely that a reflexologist would agree to treat a child under these circumstances, as a doctor's referral should always be sought.

PROHIBITED APPELLATION

This makes it a criminal offence for anyone who does not hold the relevant qualification to use any of the following titles: chemist, chiropodist, dental practitioner, dentist, dietician, doctor, druggist, general practitioner, medical laboratory technician, midwife, nurse, occupational therapist, optician, orthoptist, pharmacist, physiotherapist, radiographer, remedial gymnast, surgeon, veterinary practitioner, veterinary surgeon.

Relevance to reflexologists

A professional reflexologist would not claim to hold qualifications they did not possess.

PROHIBITED FUNCTIONS

It is also a criminal offence for unqualified persons to perform certain specified functions in the field of medicine: the practice of dentistry, midwifery, veterinary surgery or the treatment of venereal disease.

Relevance to reflexologists

A professional reflexologist would not perform such functions.

FRAUDULENT MEDIUMSHIP

The law provides that anyone who:

a) with intent to deceive purports to act as a spiritualistic medium or to exercise any power of telepathy, clairvoyance or other similar powers or

b) in purporting to act as a spiritualistic medium, or to exercise the powers mentioned in a) above, uses any fraudulent device is guilty of an offence.

Relevance to reflexologists

It is acceptable for a reflexologist to feel that a healing energy is used during the treatment process, but the reflexologist should not interpret this as any form of mediumship or imply that this forms part of the treatment, and certainly not use it in a deceptive or manipulative way.

ORAL REMEDIES

Medicines are termed medical products in the Medicines Act 1968. A medical product is defined as meaning any substance supplied for use by being administered to a human being for a medicinal purpose. It therefore includes not only allopathic medicines but also substances such as naturopathic remedies, the Bach remedies, vitamins, bio-chemic tissue salts etc.

Under the Act any practitioner who supplies oral remedies needs a licence *unless he passes on to his patients the remedies he obtains from his supplier in the unopened containers in which he supplies them.* In these cases no licence is required provided the *product supplier* holds a product licence covering the remedy in question.

A practitioner who obtains remedies in bulk and distributes small quantities to different patients will need a licence authorising the assembly of medicinal products.

Such a licence can be obtained by completing application form MAC14B from the Department of Health Medicine Control Agency, Market Towers, 1 Nine Elms Lane, London SW8 5NQ.

Relevance to reflexologists

A reflexologist should not prescribe or give advice on remedies or other medicines unless qualified to do so, and then it should be made clear that this does not form part of the reflexology treatment.

FALSE AND MISLEADING STATEMENTS

Under the Trade Descriptions Act 1968 any statement about the properties of goods or the nature of services offered which is false, misleading or inaccurate can give rise to prosecution.

The main importance of this Act for practitioners lies in the provision concerning false statements as to services. This includes false statements about the effect of the treatment.

Under the 1967 Misrepresentations Act a patient who engages the services of a practitioner and pays a fee for treatment which proves unsuccessful could recover these fees (and other expenses) as damages for breach of contract if he could show that he was induced to engage the practitioner's services by means of a misrepresentation made by the practitioner about the efficacy of the treatment.

Relevance to reflexologists

A practitioner should not claim to cure or diagnose or make any statement about qualifications and experience unless it is true and it can be proved to be true.

ADVERTISING

The law makes it an offence to take part in the publication of any advert referring to any article of any description in terms which are calculated to lead to the use of that article for the purpose of treating human beings for any of the following diseases: Bright's disease, glaucoma, cataract, locomotor ataxy, diabetes paralysis, epilepsy or fits, tuberculosis.

It is also an offence to publish any advert that:

a)   offers to treat or prescribe a remedy or advice for cancer, or

b)   refers to any article in terms calculated to lead to its use in the treatment of cancer.

The law does not prevent treating patients with the above diseases – in each case it is the advertising of a cure or treatment that is an offence.

Relevance to reflexologists:

A professional reflexologist will not claim to cure or diagnose specific ailments.

PROFESSIONAL NEGLIGENCE

The meaning of this in law is, broadly, that in his contracts with other citizens a person must have a certain regard for their interests and that, if through some act or omission committed without due regard, that other person sustains injury, he is able to pay damages as monetary redress for the injury inflicted.

Professional negligence is not merely being wrong – it is either the lack of the requisite knowledge and skill to undertake the case at all, or else, while possessing the necessary knowledge and skill, failure to apply it properly.

A person cannot be held responsible for failing to exercise a skill that he does not either express, or imply to claim to possess. It is, therefore, essential that practitioners avoid being judged by standards that do not properly apply to them. Whenever the question arises practitioners should make it clear that they are not doctors, that they do not hold a qualification recognised by law, and they do not claim to possess the same knowledge or exercise the same skill as doctors.

Relevance to reflexologists

To protect against claims of professional negligence the practitioner should know when a case is beyond the scope of their particular skill. It then becomes their duty to refer to a more skilful person or to take steps to ensure that the patient no longer relies implicitly on their skill alone. Practitioners should be aware of the limits of their capacity. Insurance should also be obtained.

PREMISES

When carrying out a trade or profession from any premises an individual must ensure that their working conditions and facilities to which members of the public have access are suitable and comply with all legislation.

Relevance to reflexologists

Ensure that premises are adequate under health and safety regulations. In general a practitioner must ensure that everything 'reasonably practicable' has been done to ensure the safety of clients. It is the 'reasonable' that is important and is usually interpreted as having taken all steps that a sensible person would have taken to avoid hazards and dangers. The practitioner can do this by carrying out a risk assessment. This means a list of things that have been thought about and checked, for example, trip hazards, safety of equipment used etc.

If working from retail premises then matters such as fire regulations may also have to be taken into account.

INSURANCE

All reflexologists should ensure that they have insurance that covers professional negligence. Failure to do so would not only result in disciplinary procedures from the membership organisation to which the reflexologist belongs but also, should a case be successful, in the reflexologist having to meet the costs and financial redress themselves. Insurance is discussed in a later chapter.

Task 73 • a) i) What do you understand by the term professional negligence?
  ii) State two ways in which can you safeguard yourself from possible claims of professional negligence.
  b) i) What is the main provision of the Trade Descriptions Act 1968?
  ii) Explain the importance of this to practitioners.
  c) In law, describe what is meant by the term prohibited appellation and give two examples.

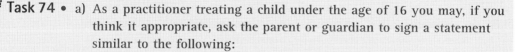

Task 74 • a) As a practitioner treating a child under the age of 16 you may, if you think it appropriate, ask the parent or guardian to sign a statement similar to the following:

I have been warned by....................................that according to the law I should consult a doctor concerning the health of my child.

Name of child............................... Signed.........................Parent or Guardian

Signed by Witness...

Explain why, in terms of the law, you would ask for such a statement

  b) Give three examples of diseases that it would be prohibited to advertise treatment for under the following legislation:

The law makes it an offence to take part in any publication or any advert referring to any article or any description in terms which are calculated to lead to the use of that article for the purpose of treating human beings for the following diseases . . .

  c) The law lists prohibited functions, which are certain specified functions within the field of medicine that unqualified persons are forbidden to perform. State two of these prohibited functions.

'SPECIAL TREATMENT' LICENCES – LOCAL COUNCIL REGULATIONS

As well as the above laws the reflexologist will also have to take into account local laws (by-laws) set up by local councils/authorities. Most local councils regulate the practice of massage and 'special treatment' through such local by-laws or council acts. The exact regulations depend very much on the local council involved and vary from stringent to non-existent, with the level of enforcement being just as variable.

Each council may have different conditions attached to the granting of a licence, often called the Standard Conditions Applied to Licences – these conditions set out what can and cannot be undertaken at the 'licensed' premises. Reflexologists may be exempt from the need to obtain a licence by virtue of their membership to the Association of Reflexologists or other reflexology association. A licence may also not be needed if only home visits are performed. For example London Local Authorities who subscribe to the 'London Local Authorities Act 1991 Part II S1–(1) list several exemptions from the need to obtain a licence, one of which is:

'Any bona fide member of an approved body of health practitioners which has given notice in writing to this council that it

a) *has a register of members;*

b) *requires as qualification for membership qualifications by way of training for, and experience of, the therapy concerned;*

c) *requires its members to hold professional indemnity insurance;*

d) *subjects its members to a code of conduct and ethics, including a prohibition of immoral conduct in the course of their practice; and*

e) *provides procedures for disciplinary proceedings in respect of its members.'*

LICENCE PROCEDURE AND APPLICATION

To ascertain whether a licence is required contact the council's Environmental Health department. This department should send an information pack explaining its licence procedures and listing any exemptions, if you belong to a professional reflexology organisation with a satisfactory code of ethics (see Chapter 23 for an explanation of the code of ethics). Should you need to apply for a licence you will be required to fill in an application form, the exact format of which may vary from authority to authority. A licence fee will be due; again the cost of varies from council to council.

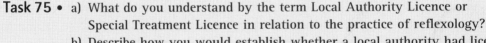

Task 75 • a) What do you understand by the term Local Authority Licence or Special Treatment Licence in relation to the practice of reflexology?
b) Describe how you would establish whether a local authority had licence requirements.

CHAPTER 27

Bookkeeping, tax and accounts

Important note:

This chapter relates to the UK only. Other countries, regions and states may have different legislation. Contact the relevant authorities in the country or region where you live, if outside the UK.

If you intend to offer reflexology for profit or gain rather than just as a part-time interest for use on family and friends then you will need to be registered for tax purposes.

The information in this chapter is intended as a basic guide. It is *not* an exhaustive list of requirements and is not a substitute for the services of a qualified accountant, whom you should engage as soon as funds allow – particularly if your tax matters are complicated and involve large amounts of capital or investment in property/lease purchase etc. Accountant's fees are tax deductible!

INCOME TAX

Each individual is entitled to a personal allowance. This is the amount of money you can earn before paying tax. For example in 2001/2002 the basic single person's allowance for those born after 5 April 1927 was £4,535. Each year it usually increases by the inflation rate. There are different allowances for married couples and additional personal allowances in certain other circumstances. The Inland Revenue can issue a notice of coding which shows the amount of money you can earn before paying tax, based on your own personal circumstances.

Taxable income is divided into rate bands, which are chargeable at different percentages. For example the rates for 2000/2001 were:

Basic rates	Higher rate
10% on the first £1,880 of taxable income	
22% on the next £27,519 of taxable income	40% over £29,400

If you are working for an employer and running your business part-time you will still need to keep accounts and pay tax on your part-time earnings. It is likely that your PAYE (pay as you earn) under your employer will be affected.

NATIONAL INSURANCE

You are also liable to pay National Insurance contributions, which represent each person's contribution to unemployment benefit, sickness benefit, invalidity benefit and state pensions. Flat rate class 2 contributions are payable by all self-employed persons. If your earnings fall below the class 2 contribution level you may opt to apply for a small earnings exemption so that payments are halted, or you may continue to pay to protect your benefits.

Class 4 contributions may also be payable if all your profits as an individual, when added together, come to more than a set amount. The class 4 contributions are calculated as a percentage of profits that fall between an upper and lower limit.

Task 76 • a) What do you understand by the following terms:
　　　　 i) National Insurance
　　　　 ii) tax allowance?
　　　 b) What information would a notice of coding give you?
　　　 c) If, as a self-employed practitioner, your earnings fall below the Class 2 National Insurance contributions level, what are your two options?

HOW TO KEEP BASIC ACCOUNTS

The tax year (financial year) runs from 1 April–31 March. Your accounts can be made up yearly from the start date of your business or you may have a short first year to bring the accounts into line with the financial year.

Every year you must fill in a *self-assessment tax return* form which will enable you to calculate the amount of tax you owe in a financial year. You must then pay this amount in two instalments the following January and July. Failure to submit a tax return or pay tax bills results in fines and interest charges.

The tax return requires details of everything earnt and spent against the business for the year in question. The return has a section where you can calculate your own tax or it can be calculated for you by the taxman, depending on when you submit the return.

There are two things everybody must do:

1. Let the tax man know if you need a tax return – for instance if you have received new income or changed circumstances tell the tax man within six months of the end of the tax year in which the new circumstances apply. If you start in self-employment notify the Inland Revenue via your local tax office.

2. Keep records of income and expenditure. This includes all receipts/invoices/bank statements/paying-in books etc.

The three main types of information you will need to keep are:

1. All income.

2. All deductible expenses.

3. Money drawn for your own use.

ALL INCOME

This means any money received in connection with the business; for example:

*   Treatment charges

*   Sale of stock (creams, lotions etc.)

*   Lecture fees

*   Grants/loans etc.

Also keep a copy of all receipts you issue, and do not discard previous years' appointment diaries.

ALL DEDUCTIBLE EXPENSES

Deductible expenses are those genuinely incurred in connection with the operation of your business. The cost of these expenses is offset against any income before arriving at the net profit. It is important, therefore, to ensure you make full use of your allowable expenses. The tax man has a full list of elements that are allowed under this category but below are the main items of expenditure which, as a reflexologist, you may incur as allowable expenses:

Remember, *keep all receipts and invoices.*

PURCHASE OF BUSINESS STOCK

All items that you have purchased to undertake your profession and which, generally speaking, can be used up or sold on within the tax year. e.g. talc and oils for feet, towels, couch roll, posters, etc.

CAPITAL ALLOWANCES

Capital equipment is, broadly speaking, anything than can't be used up within a year of purchase, e.g. couch, computers etc. Capital equipment cannot be treated as a business expense for the year in which you buy it, but you may be able to claim capital allowances instead. This spreads the tax relief over a number of years by allowing a percentage value each year.

RENT/RATES

Rent paid for a treatment room in a clinic.

If you have set aside a room in your house exclusively for business purposes you may claim a proportion of the overall rent and maintenance of the property to offset against profits. However, Be careful! If you do decide to set aside a room in your house exclusively for business purposes (generally considered to be more than ten per cent of the area) you may become liable to pay business rates and Capital Gains tax on the proceeds of the sale of your home.

A dual use room – i.e. some business and some private use – will not attract Capital Gains tax and will still allow a proportion of light and heating costs to be offset.

TELEPHONE

All your bills may be included if you have a separate business line. If you use your domestic number you may claim a percentage of the overall bill.

OTHER ITEMS

Insurance, subscriptions, training (your payments for professional insurance and membership of professional bodies and associations). Postage, printing and stationery, repairs and renewals, motor expenses (mileage in connection with the business), cleaning, protective clothing, travelling, pension contributions, depreciation on certain items.

ALL MONEY DRAWN FOR SELF

Money drawn out of the business for your personal use or use for something not connected with the business.

WEEKLY ACCOUNTS

From the records kept in 1, 2 and 3 above it is essential that weekly accounts are made in order for the yearly tax return to be submitted to the tax man. It may be that you keep weekly accounts yourself that you then give to your accountant to compile the accounts for tax return purposes.

Weekly **outgoings**

Use headings that match your outgoings – have as many or as few as needed

Week	Business stock	Printing and stationery	Adverts and publicity	Telephone	Insurance and professional memberships	Clinic rental	Postage
1. (1–7 April)	120	500	50		140	120	10
2. (8–14 April)	10		50			120	5
3. (15–21 April)	25	25	50	120		120	12
TOTALS	155	525	150	120	140	360	27

Use a line for each week, e.g. 1–52

Give a total for each heading – monthly total are probably best, which can then be added to make a yearly total

Weekly **income**

Week	Treatments	Lectures	Sale of stock
1. (1–7 April)	220	75	25
2. (8–14 April)	350		15
3. (15–21 April)	350	25	5
TOTALS	920	100	45

Figure 19 Example of a weekly accounting record

Figure 19 suggests how to keep weekly records. This is based on the average requirements of a reflexologist but may not cater for all possible areas of expenditure and income. There are also many ready-made account books, which are relatively simple to keep and easily understood by an accountant making up your end of year accounts.

Figure 20 shows a suggested income and expenditure account, which could be used to help fill in the tax return. It is recommended that an accountant be involved in the compilation of the tax return, but if your turnover is low and your tax affairs uncomplicated then it is possible to do it yourself. Once again this is a basic submission and may not cater for all possible areas of income and expenditure. The example uses the figures from Figure 19 as an illustration of how the weekly record can be used to compile an end of year account.

The net profit is calculated by taking the expenditure figure from the income figure. In this example there would be no tax to pay on the net profit as it is below the personal tax allowance threshold.

If your annual turnover is less than £15,000 you have the option to supply the tax man with three line accounts on your tax return – showing turnover, expenditure and profit. You must still keep detailed records.

Income and expenditure account for Mr B Toe, year ending 31 March 2003

Income		
Treatments	920	
Lectures	100	
Sale of stock	45	
TOTAL		1,065

Expenditure		
Business stock	155	
Printing and stationery	25	
Adverts and publicity	150	
Telephone	120	
Insurance and professional memberships	140	
Clinic rental	360	
Postage	27	
TOTAL		977

Net profit	88

Figure 20 Example of a yearly accounting return

Figure 21 shows a bank account report. This is a useful way of monitoring all transactions through your business bank account. It can also be checked against your bank statement, which gives details of all amounts paid in or drawn out of the account, together with a balance at a particular date – usually monthly. It is for your own records, and is not required as part of the tax return. This type of report will help keep track of the day-to-day monies going in and out of your account, and so make sure you know exactly what money you have in the bank at any given time. It will also help to check your monthly bank statements against this record to ensure there have been no mistakes. It is not a substitute for the weekly records as shown in Figure 19 but an additional aid for viewing the state of your business.

VAT

Value Added Tax is a 17.5 per cent charge on goods and services, if the turnover of a business is above a certain level. Turnover means the amount of money made by the business *before* anything is deducted for expenses. The percentage charge for VAT and the turnover level may vary each year according to the chancellor's budget. In 2001/2002 it is 17.5 per cent for turnover in excess of £54,000. In practical terms this means that most reflexologists will not have to register for VAT or charge it on their services. It does also mean, however, that VAT cannot be reclaimed on items bought. Since a reflexologist does not buy many large VAT – inclusive items this is not a significant issue, and it is far better to remain outside the VAT system, in terms of extra paperwork and returns, unless

Date	Spent	Cheque number	Received	Paying in slip/receipt number	Balance
3/4/2003			600	001 – Opening loan	600
4/4/2003	150	00001 – Treatment chair			450
5/4/2003	20	00002 – Various stock items			430
10/4/2003	50	0003 –Clinic rent			380
10/4/2003			45	002 – Treatment	425
12/4/2003			45	003 – Treatment	470
12/4/2003	Current bank balance				**470**

Figure 21 Example of a bank account report

there is an overriding reason to register. It is possible to register voluntarily with a turnover of less than the VAT limit, but seek professional accountancy advice before doing so.

TROUBLE WITH TAX?

It goes without saying that you should always be honest with your tax affairs. Do not attempt to hide income or falsify records.

The Inland Revenue has its own advice lines where small business can get answers to general tax enquiries. The numbers are listed in the phone book under Inland Revenue. There is also a general help line for self-assessment queries (0845 9000 444) and a very useful website at www.inlandrevenue.gov.uk. It is also possible to submit tax returns on-line.

Every year a random sample of businesses is selected for enquiry, which could mean anything from just seeking confirmation of one particular figure on your tax return to a detailed investigation of all your business records and other tax affairs. It is possible to take out a special form of business insurance that will provide representations to the revenue on your behalf, should you become the subject of a detailed investigation, or provide money to cover accountant's fees.

Task 77 • a) Give two possible tax effects of using a room in your home exclusively for business.

b) What information does a bank statement give you?

c) As a self-employed person you are required to keep certain records for accounting purposes. Give three of the categories of information that must be kept.

d) What do you understand by the following terms:
   i) VAT
   ii) net profit?

CHAPTER 28

Insurance

Every reflexologist must ensure that they have adequate insurance for the practice of their profession. There are two essential elements that should be present in any insurance scheme: public liability and professional indemnity.

PUBLIC LIABILITY

This covers the practitioner for accidents occurring to clients before, during or immediately after treatment, for example tripping over your carpet, falling down the stairs or off the couch etc. The cover provided should be at least to the value of £1,000,000. This means if you are successfully sued by a third party the insurance company will pay out up to this amount.

Caution: Always read the small print of insurance policies to make sure that they actually cover what you think they cover i.e. that there are no major exemptions hidden away such as 'not covered if treating in premises other than the main practice'.

PROFESSIONAL INDEMNITY

This covers the practitioner for damage to clients caused by the treatment itself. It as also known as malpractice insurance. Many such policies are often for one particular treatment only so if you are qualified in and practice more than reflexology, you may need another policy to cover you or to extend the current policy to include other therapies.

Note: This type of cover is sometimes attached to public liability insurance with various exemptions such as 'sports injuries only' or 'not including psychological damage'.

Many policies will also offer additional cover for specific areas, for example accidental damage to equipment or cover for selling oils/lotions made up by the practitioner (product insurance).

The area of practitioner insurance is still expanding and many other options may be available in the future. Whatever policies you choose always ensure that at public liability and professional indemnity are covered.

OTHER INSURANCE ISSUES

If working from home and you have a lease then you must ensure that there are no restrictive clauses in it that prevent conducting a business from the premises. If there are it is likely that any public and professional liability insurance will be invalidated.

If travelling to treat clients then you should ensure that your car insurance covers you for travel to and from more than one place of work (sometimes known as class 1 insurance).

It may also be worth considering insurance policies that pay out if you are incapacitated and unable to work for a long period, or insurance for your hands. There are many different types of policies covering this area and it is best to seek the advice of an independent financial advisor (IFA) before making a final decision.

 Task 78 • a) What are the names of the two essential types of insurance a practitioner should have before treating the public? Explain the purpose of each.

b) Besides the above, name two other types of insurance that may be needed by a reflexologist.

FINALLY – *DON'T WORRY!*

In practice it is extremely rare to be sued for malpractice or have a claim made against you for an unforeseen accident but it is essential that you are covered in order to sleep well at night!

CHAPTER 29

Taking bookings and charging for treatments

Once you have released your publicity and marketing it is very important to be ready to take bookings from clients. Answering the telephone is the first obvious area to think about. This initial contact is the first impression a client gets of you and your practice.

HOW WILL YOU ANSWER CALLS?

Just answering with 'Hello?' will cause confusion for the client. They will not be sure if they have the right number and will then have to ask further questions to establish your identity. This is not a good first impression.

If you have only one telephone line for business and personal use then answer the phone with your name – this will sound more professional to prospective clients and your friends and family will get used to it.

Some telephone companies offer a service where you can have a second telephone number attached to a single line – this rings with a different tone. This option is less expensive than a second line and alerts you to a reflexology call which you can then answer with your practice name and be ready to take further details. Other householders will also know that the call is for you. A second line is the other option, which is the most expensive but gives you the most control over handling calls. It is also fully deductible against tax.

Once you have decided which option you prefer you will need to consider how best to ensure that you do not miss business calls. Clients may ring at times when you are treating or out. An answering machine will enable you to follow up missed calls – again make sure the message is appropriate for potential reflexology clients. In addition some telephone companies offer a service that allows callers to leave a message if the line is busy.

HOW WILL YOU TAKE BOOKINGS?

Over time you will become more experienced in handling clients' initial enquiries and bookings, indeed you may already have experience when seeing clients for your practice treatments. The following is a suggested checklist for the initial client booking. You may wish to adapt it to suit your approach, but it is a very good idea to have something like it in the front of your appointment diary, so that you remember in the early stages to ask all the relevant questions. It is particularly important to have it with your appointment diary, as this is the first place you will look when making bookings.

BOOKING CHECKLIST – FIRST TIME CLIENT

Question/action	Reason
How did you hear about me?	Establishes if client is from recommendation or from publicity. Helps identify what sources of publicity are working for you. Helps you decide if you need to ask *further personal safety questions* – see Chapter 24 for a list of these questions.
Ask further personal safety questions if appropriate	Helps to ensure the client is genuine. See Chapter 24 for a list of personal safety questions.
Have you had reflexology before?	Establishes if the caller needs to have reflexology explained. If so give a very brief description and tell them what to expect during a treatment. Tell them what qualification you hold. Also explain that a medical history will be taken on the first appointment.
Are you suffering from thrombosis or phlebitis?	Establishes if a major contraindication is present – in which case a treatment should not be undertaken.
What is your main health problem? How long have you had this condition? Who have you seen previously for this condition? What results have you had under previous care?	These questions are designed to be general, so as not to subject the client to an interrogation, but give you valuable information in order to judge the urgency of the case. For example a client may phone to demand an appointment immediately because they are in pain. Research shows that people seeking alternative/complementary advice have been unwell anywhere from one to 31 years. Suddenly something moves them to phone for an appointment and demand to see someone straight away. These basic questions will help you to decide if and when you can see them and to avoid unnecessary disruption of your schedule. It will also help you to research the condition, if it is not already known to you.

Question/action	Reason
Arrange an appointment date and time. Inform of the length of time the treatment will take. Write in appointment diary along with client contact details.	Agrees a mutually convenient time for both client and practitioner.
State fee and how payment will be accepted. State cancellation policy (if you have one).	Establishes that payment will be due from the client and how they can pay. Client knows that an amount will be due if appointment is cancelled within 24 hours (or other terms and conditions if you have a cancellation policy).
Give address details for treatment or establish details for home visit	Client knows where to come or practitioner knows where to travel. If visiting the client remember the personal safety questions in Chapter 24.
Repeat appointment details	Clarifies arrangements
Ask if client has any other questions	Gives client opportunity to clarify anything that was not clear.
Finish call with further reminder of date and time of appointment	Finalises conversation. Reinforces treatment arrangements.
Check date and time in appointment diary	To confirm your own administrative records.
Make a note in appointment diary in the week before the appointment to send postal confirmation. Make another note in the appointment diary the day before the treatment to phone and remind client.	Lessens chance of client forgetting. Confirms client has given correct personal details – see personal safety questions in Chapter 24.

Remember to keep a checklist like this with your appointment diary to ensure you remember everything involved in taking a booking from a first time client.

Task 79 • List what you consider to be five essential questions you would ask a first time client when taking a booking over the telephone.

CHARGING FOR TREATMENT

Many practitioners often find it difficult to ask for payment. Do not confuse the client's inconvenience of paying for an inability to pay. Most clients have the ability to pay but sometimes find it more convenient to spend their money on clothes, holidays and anything else apart from health care.

If your practice is run in a sloppy haphazard fashion and the layout is unprofessional you will run the risk of attracting the type of patient who resents paying. If, however, you are running a professional businesslike practice and explain to new clients *before* treatment the fees involved and the methods of payment you should have no trouble extracting the money at the end of a session. If you still feel awkward asking for payment remember that you are a qualified professional providing an individual and caring service – you deserve to be paid!

TIME SLOTS

Allow an interval between clients in order to reset the room and give yourself a slight rest. As you gain more experience you will be able to time your treatments accurately and thus lessen the intervals but initially allow plenty of time between clients in case you overrun.

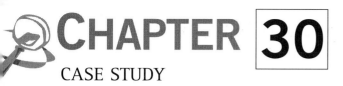

CHAPTER 30

CASE STUDY

CASE STUDIES FROM THE AUTHOR'S CLINIC

It is always useful to share case studies and treatment histories, as it can help with the treatment of other clients with similar presenting conditions.

The following chapters contain some of my own clients' case studies.

To prepare a first time client for a hands-on treatment I always give a brief description of what I am going to do and how the client is likely to feel. Remember this may be the first time the client has received any form of complementary treatment. I always tell my students to inform the client that it is all right to relax, which may cause them to fall asleep. It is also okay to pause the session if the client needs a bathroom break. It may be a good idea to see if the client wants to use your facilities before you commence the treatment.

I have also had clients apologise for falling asleep, though they never apologise in future sessions as I have explained to them that it is their time. They should be encouraged to use it to sleep, laugh, snore, drift in and out of a deeply relaxed state, use the time to let go and be recharged and rebalanced.

When I have finished the client consultation and am about to inspect the condition of the client's feet, I ask the client to stand in bare feet so that it is easier to check for varicose veins. If the client's legs are elevated varicose veins may not be as obvious. If the client has this condition or broken thread veins then I work lightly around these areas. Remember: never work directly over varicose veins. I can also check for condition of the arch of the foot, useful if they have a high arch, as when I come to treat the spine reflexes I will know to work a little higher into this area. Conversely I will know to work lower in the case of a dropped arch.

Once the client is on the couch or treatment chair I make sure they are comfortable with neck supported and that the mid and lower back are correctly positioned, with a pillow for support, under the knees. If I am working on a couch I check regularly for client back discomfort. Clients often find it more comfortable to be lying flat, rather than propped up, with plenty of extra support under the knees. It is still possible to see the client if they are lying down. I always prefer to use a treatment chair if possible, as I have found it much better for client comfort.

Before starting the treatment I always wipe the feet over with a moistened tissue to clean and refresh them. Then I apply a little powder over the feet and massage this in, to aid grip when working the reflex points. If you do not wish to use standard talcum powder there are several alternatives on the market, which give the same effect but are talc-free. Some practitioners prefer to use cream and others nothing. I would suggest you use whichever suits you best.

CASE STUDY A – FEMALE CLIENT AGED 35

This client first came to me when I was running a clinic at a health club. Her presenting complaint was migraine, from which she had been suffering for several months, only using medication when she had to.

After taking a full medical history and looking at the client's lifestyle I could see there were a number of problem areas. Her work was high powered and stressful and also involved a lot of travel. Her health had been good until a few years ago when she had suffered for several weeks in February with flu. She took just ten days off work during this period and returned while still unwell (a regular pattern with young high earners – deadlines first, health second, happiness third). I felt she had not listened to her body and may have developed a post viral syndrome, only resting when not working. She now wanted a quick fix. I think migraine was her body's last scream for help.

I knew I would have to treat the migraine first, in order that she stayed the distance for further treatments, which could then address the deeper issues. I worked deeply to all reflexes with particular attention to head, neck, brain, occipital, balance, spine and adrenals. This would help balance the nervous system, muscular and skeletal systems and have a positive pain-relieving effect.

The client found great sensitivity in all neck reflexes, the adrenals and cervical spine. I felt I needed to treat with deep pressure to enable the client to let go and relax more, making her feel confident that I was doing the work! She did not relax until I was on the left foot, but she was sleeping by the end of the treatment. I left her to rest for a further ten minutes. On waking she said she felt extremely heavy and tired and her head pain had reduced to a dull ache. I booked in a follow-up treatment in five days.

When the client returned she reported feeling tired since the last session. She had felt less tense and had not had a migraine, but a dull ache for the last several days. She felt this was positive.

I explained to the client that her job sounded like it was not going to change and that to get her back on the road to optimum health we needed to be more intensive with the treatments. I suggested two to three treatments a week, for the first two weeks, then to re-evaluate. She said she could manage this, but only with evening appointments, so I recommended straight from work to the couch!

For the second treatment I repeated the strategy of the first as I felt she had responded very well. I did give some extra work to the spleen for energy regeneration. I worked this point at least ten times, with a firm pressure. She slept on and off during the whole treatment.

When I triggered the heart reflex she woke up immediately saying it felt like an electric shock. To me this meant the client was having difficulty letting go of emotions that manifested themselves physically and resulted in a tightness in the chest area. I worked this area with less pressure and reassured her that her reaction was normal for the treatment process. It later emerged that she had forgotten to tell me she suffered from palpitations several years previously over a six-month period, which stopped only once she had been promoted at work. I fed back what she had said and she realised that her strong perfectionist streak had obviously made her strive towards the promotion with the consequent stress of the palpitations. I thought this justified more work on the heart reflex, in order to combat the mental and emotional stress of perfectionism! I applied medium pressure, holding and rotating for at least two minutes, then repeating. The client also reported that the colon was sensitive on the left foot. This told me we needed to spend more time concentrating on elimination and detoxing. I felt sensitivity in the spinal lumbar region, mainly L3 and L4. As she reported no lower back pain I felt this was more likely to do with circulation in her legs. During the treatment she reported that she would often spend hours working on her computer at home in the evenings. I suggested that she take regular five-minute breaks from this work in order to stretch and walk up and down to assist peripheral circulation and relieve back stiffness. The client was so much more relaxed during the treatment, drifting in and out of sleep.

I saw her four days later for the third treatment when she reported more improvement but still felt tired. I suggested that after this treatment she go straight home for an early night, after a light snack and plenty of water. I gave extra work to the endocrine system to help with emotional and physical balance. I also worked for longer on the excretory system i.e. the liver, gall bladder, kidneys, intestines, bladder and lymphs to help with detoxification and boost the immune system. The liver was the most sensitive of these points, so I re-worked it with ten more pressure, rotate and release movements. I did the same for the spleen. I arranged to see the client again in five days.

On the fourth treatment she looked brighter and appeared to have more energy. She reported feeling that she had more energy and had not had a headache or migraine since the last treatment. I was convinced the extra work I had performed on the excretory system had really made a difference and decided to repeat my focus on these areas during the treatment. I also added deeper and extra work to the spinal reflexes, across the spine as well as down, in order to provide extra stimulation to the nerves that branch from the spine to the internal organs. I also reminded her of the no work rule after the nights of her treatment, as I was convinced this also made a big difference to her condition and gave the treatment time to work.

A week later I saw her for the fifth time and suggested that I show her some reflex points on the hands. I find this helps the client to take some responsibility for the treatment process, and gets them involved in their own health and well-being. I showed her the reflex points before the treatment, as afterwards the client is too relaxed to be able to concentrate and retain the information. I showed her the following hand reflexes: solar plexus (to be worked seven times on each hand), gall bladder, liver, kidneys, lymph, spleen, colon and spine, with extra attention to the cervical spine. I was sure this was the region that caused most of the tightness and stress thus causing the headaches and migraines. I suggested she complete the mini hand work-out by returning to the solar plexus. I wrote down the sequence and suggested she performed it several times a week for about 15 minutes each time. I also supplied her with a copy of the video, showing the hand reflexology points – so she had no excuses!

Not all clients need homework but this one was doing so well I knew that when she came to completing her course of treatments she may well lapse, so self-treatment was perfect for her busy lifestyle.

Several more sessions followed, reduced to once every two weeks, then once a month. Her condition remained improved and I found myself concentrating more on the spine and heart with each treatment, as this seemed to reinforce the improvements in her condition and improve the relaxing effect of the treatment. I also became more focused on the excretory organs to help with elimination of toxins. On more than one occasion during the final few treatments she commented that she felt more in control of her life and had started to put herself first on several occasions! I couldn't have asked for more evidence that my treatment plan was working, and that we had both succeeded in improving her quality of life.

It is important to remember that putting time aside for oneself is not an act of selfishness, but one of self-preservation. By looking after number one its then possible to support, care for, help and love numbers two three and four, whether they be friends, children, lovers or work!

CASE STUDY B – FEMALE CLIENT AGED 80

This lady is one of the many older clients I treat. She first came to see me ten years ago just before her seventieth birthday and hasn't stopped since!

I first saw her while working at a podiatrist clinic. A family member or friend had recommended her, and as she was a regular at the clinic it was convenient to see me also. She had never experienced a complementary treatment, so after a brief chat about what to expect from the treatment I went on to take a full medical history.

She had lower back problems and, although not in constant pain, she felt it was a real nuisance. There were also varicose veins on the backs of both legs, although they did not extend to the feet. She was also under treatment for leukaemia with the local hospital. This was under control and there were regular check-ups to monitor her blood count. She had checked with her consultant who had no objections to her receiving a reflexology treatment.

Her first sessions were general treatments to all reflex areas so that I could get her used to the treatment and record areas of sensitivity. Most sensitive areas were the neck, spine, pituitary and intestine. She reported sleeping better after the sessions and really enjoyed receiving them.

At the third session she reported much improvement in the back pain, but that there was still a lack of mobility in the area. I took this as an encouraging sign as it seemed to indicate a regression of the symptoms to an earlier stage. With more work I felt this could regress further resulting in greater mobility. There was still sensitivity in the neck, head and sinus reflexes on both feet, but she did not report any headaches or sinus problems. Overall her attitude towards the treatment had become very positive, she believed it would really help her. Other areas of sensitivity were the knee, hip and lower back, with the main sensitivity in the hip reflex. I felt it was important therefore to give extra work to the skeletal muscular system, in particular the spine and hip reflexes.

As a general note it can be tempting to wrap older clients in 'cotton wool', treating them too gently and not allowing a growth in their treatment. Although there are times when lighter and shorter treatments are necessary, this is not always the case and the reflexologist should not be put off pursuing a vigorous treatment programme on an elderly client if and when the time is right.

She would often report after subsequent treatments that her legs felt lighter and that the hot and aching feelings that she often experienced due to the varicose veins had subsided considerably.

During the following two treatments as well as maintaining pressure on the muscular and skeletal systems I also focused more on the circulatory system. I paid extra attention to the heart, diaphragm, liver and lungs. I also gave extra work to the lumbar vertebrae to help with the circulation to the legs.

The colon was sensitive on the left foot during these sessions and the client reported mild constipation. I worked the colon and colon helper area for longer and went back to the liver in order to help with elimination. I also suggested that she drink more water, as mild dehydration can often contribute towards constipation.

At the next session she reported that her constipation had cleared.

During the treatment programme she had regular blood tests in order that her consultant could monitor the leukaemia. It was noted that her white blood count was down, which was a very positive sign.

She also had a slightly dropped arch for which she had seen a podiatrist who had recommended orthotics (an insert into the shoe, which helps support the foot). I suggested that she wear the orthotic and that when she was buying shoes she made sure that they had a good, supportive instep. I even managed to get her to buy a pair of trainers, which helped support her foot.

By the eighth session she had reported that her back stiffness had eased significantly and that she was able to walk much further than she had in years. I continued, however, to detect sensitivity within the lumbar reflexes.

I continued to see this client for sustaining treatments on a monthly or bi-monthly basis. She continues to see me because she really believes that the treatments added significantly to her ability to fight back against her condition and also give her an extra energy boost. From my point of view she has become one of my favourite regulars, as she is always so positive and determined to work with me in getting the most from the therapy.

CASE STUDY C – FEMALE AGED 41

This woman came to me on the recommendation of another client, whom I had treated for many years as well as her children and grandchildren, so her expectations were high. This was her first encounter with complementary therapies. She came from a medical background, being a nurse. After first meeting me she confessed that she had thought that all complementary therapists were 'way out', with men in ponytails greeting their clients in brown sandals! She had a plan to excuse herself to feed the parking meter and never return if her suspicions were correct. Thankfully her preconceptions were not founded, as I always place great importance on a professional appearance.

Her medical history consultation showed that she had sustained a lower back injury 12 years previously, treated at the time with physiotherapy. There were no current problems resulting from this old injury. Prior to this there had been an operation on the right knee, for ligament reconstruction, which was successful, although there were occasional mild aches and pains in this area. There was a family history of high blood pressure.

Her current presenting condition was one of extreme stress, which had led to anxiety and depression. She had two young children, a new home (in the process of renovation), and a husband who was frequently away on business, working long hours.

It is worth noting that people in the caring professions are often great at sorting out other people's problems, whether health, emotional or friendship, but hopeless at looking after themselves. Their needs are put to the back of the queue, until they become run down, unhappy or ill. This is not always the case, but having treated many therapists, it is my experience that they help themselves only at the last minute.

This client was taking sleeping tablets and prozac, which made her feel constantly tired and run down. She also had a natural instinct to be in charge and control situations, which worked against the current feeling of hopelessness and anxiety. It seemed that she needed to hit rock bottom before she could let go, move on and rebuild.

When you are the last port of call for a client who likes to lead, is self-critical, carries everyone but lacks confidence, is anxious but craves stimulants, what do you do?

Firstly, we need to try and help them feel good about themselves. So after explaining what to expect from reflexology, I launched straight into the treatment, taking care to lower the back rest into a position that would avoid direct eye contact, while reassuring her that I could see her reactions, thus not tempting her to seize control of the situation.

I knew there would be some resistance during the first treatment and this was confirmed with only a few reflex areas showing sensitivity and the feet feeling somewhat cold and resistive to touch. I gave extra work to the endocrine system to help balance on a physical and emotional level. The left foot was a little more sensitive than the right. The left foot sensitive reflexes were the spinal reflexes, sciatic point and heart. The chest and breast areas felt resistive and tight on both feet and I felt this would be an area for extra attention in future sessions along with the heart reflex.

I saw the client again after four days and she reported not much change since the first treatment, but she did wish to commit to a course of treatments. I felt very positive about this step, and felt a great empathy with the client. She reported problems with her house renovation work and feeling very stressed so I got straight on with treatment. I spent more time on the chest, spine and heart reflexes. I felt that she was more at ease with the treatment, so I was able to increase the pressure and length of some of the treatment points in order to bring about a deeper change.

A week later she returned for a third treatment. She reported feeling better in herself since the last session. My own feelings were that the care and support involved in the treatment process were just as important as the treatment itself in aiding her recovery. This session showed the right pituitary as very sensitive, a new development. As the leader of the endocrine system this gland is vital in influencing health and stability, and its sensitivity meant I could spend extra time stimulating it, returning to it at several points during the treatment session. The left lumbar vertebrae were also all sensitive. The client reported heaviness in her legs and lower back, which tied in with the lumbar sensitivity. Some therapists also believe that sensitive lumbar reflexes reflect a client who is feeling unsupported.

On the fourth treatment session she reported facing a challenging situation since the last treatment, but felt better able to cope than ever before. I took this as an indication that the treatments were having an effect on an emotional and physical level. Both pituitary points were now sensitive along with a slight sensitivity of the spinal reflexes (greater sensitivity on the left side). The neck was moderately sensitive on both sides along with the adrenals. The sciatic was sensitive on the left side. The intestines also showed moderate sensitivity. The increase of pituitary sensitivity to both sides of the feet further indicated a rebalancing of the endocrine system. The intestine sensitivity reflected her feelings of stomach knots in difficult situations. A weakness of the muscular/skeletal system (reflected in the spine, neck and sciatic reflexes) seemed to stem from the previous old injuries so I treated this as a mildly chronic problem rather than as acute. It indicated to me that we were progressing to the core stages of the treatment.

As we progressed with further treatments it became obvious that we had reached the core stage, as she felt less reliant on medication and more able to deal with stressful situations. The regular treatments, combined with encouragement to relax during the treatments, really improved her condition. I continued extra work on the endocrine system and spinal reflexes along with a longer closing sequence to aid relaxation.

I treated this client a total of 25 times and felt that by this stage she had developed the inner resources to cope with her situation in a more balanced way, and that she was having a much better relationship with herself. I decided to treat her on a monthly basis only, as I did not want her to become too dependent on the treatment. As therapists we have to recognise that letting go of clients can be just as therapeutic as treating them. We must be able to judge when to reduce clients to a sustaining treatment, in order to maximise the benefits of the entire treatment programme.

CASE STUDY D – MALE AGED 28

This client came to me at a clinic where several different forms of complementary therapies were offered. He walked in off the street and decided that reflexology was the treatment for him, as he was on his feet all day.

The initial consultation revealed that he was a builder and worked long hours of strenuous activity, often lifting and carrying heavy materials and eating only when there was a chance. His diet consisted mainly of fast, fried food and beer! He suffered minor aches and pains due to his profession. He had, however, developed severe pain within his right wrist and elbow, which I suspected might be due to repetitive strain injury (RSI). He reported finding it very difficult to get up each morning – probably due to late-night drinking and eating sessions.

His medical history revealed that both parents were fit and well but that his father had suffered a heart attack five years previously but made a full recovery. One positive attribute this had on his health was that it had made him give up smoking. The client took very little regular exercise, apart from his work, which was more lifting and repetitive, developing certain muscles rather than exercise that was cardiovascular (strengthening the heart and circulation).

During the first treatment I recommended that he avoid the pub afterwards. I told him that unless he did this he would be throwing his money away, as he would not feel any benefit of the treatment. I felt this direct approach might get him to concur. I gave a general treatment, concentrating with extra work on the excretory system to heal, cleanse and detoxify, although amazingly these points were not overly sensitive. The spleen showed signs of sensitivity so I returned to it several times during the treatment in order to help boost his energy levels. Both shoulder reflexes were also sensitive as well as the right foot and upper arm, elbow, lower arm and wrist. I gave extra work to all these areas, working in downward and upward bites in order to help combat the pain in his wrist and elbow, which I felt may have started at the shoulder and thus made the arm more vulnerable to an RSI-type condition. I also decided to pay extra attention to the knee reflex on the right side, as this is the cross reflex to the elbow, to boost the healing potential of the treatment.

My concerns were that because of his occupation it was going to be very difficult for him to rest the affected arm, as if he did not work he did not earn money.

I mentioned to him that a high-strength Glucosamine and Chondroitin supplement tablet had helped other clients with similar muscular/skeletal conditions. A gel of the same constituents could also be purchased which could be kept in the fridge and applied morning and night to the whole of the arm and hand. (Please remember that as a reflexologist you should not prescribe or give unqualified advice, but that you could refer clients to a good health food store or pharmacy for specialist natural product advice.)

On the second treatment there was a mild improvement in his energy levels, in that he was able to get out of bed each morning with more enthusiasm. He reported that he still felt tired later in the day but felt more able to stay wake. There was no improvement in the arm condition. I repeated a similar treatment pattern to the first session, with extra attention to the shoulder, arm, elbow and wrist reflexes on both feet. He reported greater sensitivity in these areas on the right foot. I followed this with extra work on both feet to particular spinal vertebrae because of their nerve pathway links to various parts of the body, namely the sixth cervical vertebrae, which helps with neck, shoulder and arm pain, the seventh cervical which helps with shoulder and elbow pain and inflammation, and the first thoracic to help with the lower arm, wrist and hand pain. He reported the main sensitivity to be the first thoracic. I also gave further extra work the adrenal glands on both feet to encourage the body to release cortico steroids to aid with an anti-inflammatory response. The ninth thoracic vertebrae was also worked in order to help the nerve supply to the adrenals. I recommended that the client return for a further treatment in four days, rather than the usual week, as I felt we needed to provide an extra boost.

On the next visit he reported a 30 per cent improvement in the arm pain. His energy levels were also improving again, although I felt I needed to tackle the constant pain in the right arm first, which would probably result in more energy due to less pain. I concentrated this session on the vertebrae spinal reflex points, as detailed on the last session, as I felt this was the major reason for the improvement. Other main areas of sensitivity were the liver and kidneys on both feet. This was probably related to his excess alcohol consumption, which not was going to change overnight. At this point I took the decision to continue to give extra work to the reflex areas relating to his arm pain, where I could have a more immediate beneficial effect, while following up with a general detoxifying treatment for the alcohol and food habits. I further suggested that he try and swap arms throughout the day, where possible, in order to rest the affected arm.

The following session was a week later and a further improvement was noted with the pain decreased by about 50 to 60 per cent.

I felt I had managed such success in a short period of time because we had tackled the problem in the early stages, thanks to his impulse to see a reflexologist for an entirely different reason. We continued with weekly treatments for another month, by which time the pain had almost entirely vanished. Following this I reduced to monthly treatments, with the intention of diverting some of the treatment process away from the arm to a deeper detoxification and balancing treatment. This will be a much longer process, but one that will pay dividends because my client now really believes in the ability of the treatment to produce results.

CASE STUDY E – FEMALE AGED 30

This client came to me when she was seven months pregnant. It was her first pregnancy. She was in excellent health and her medical history was brief, having never had an operation or major illness. The client reported being about 3 kg overweight for the past five to seven years.

The main reason for her visit was due to fluid retention affecting her hands, fingers, ankles and legs. She reported feeling tired and 'heavy'. She also commented that so far her pregnancy had been perfect – giving her no problems apart from the above. She was very much looking forward to the birth.

I decided to treat her on a special reclining chair rather than a couch, as this would be more comfortable. It also meant the legs could be elevated, helping the lymphatic system to drain the fluid from the legs. Once she was comfortable

I started with a gentle massage of the feet and legs, always working towards the heart to encourage drainage of the lymph. I spent about five minutes on each leg with the gentle massage movements. I then began with the opening movements.

The first sensitivity of the treatment came with the cervical and neck reflexes followed by the shoulder and diaphragm. I established that she was working at home using a computer to help with her garden design business. It was her posture during the computer use that had triggered the sensitive reactions. She also commented that her business involved manual work, which could leave her hands, back and neck sore although she would always stretch these areas after work and take a hot shower to help with the stiffness.

The liver, kidney and lymph areas were also sensitive, especially around the ankle area. I worked on these a little longer and incorporated sliding and drainage movements to encourage lymph flow. She was fast asleep by the end of the treatment.

I saw the client one week later and repeated the gentle massage to the feet and lower legs before commencing the treatment. She reported that her ankles were less puffy after the previous treatment, although in a day or two the swelling had returned. I decided to give extra work to the lymph, kidney and liver areas to stimulate the excretory system. The kidney reflex was sensitive on both feet, reinforcing the need for extra work to this area. I also suggested that she try to drink at least a bottle of water a day and to drink water alongside tea and coffee. The colon area on the left foot was slightly sensitive and she mentioned that she had been suffering from slight constipation for a few days after the treatment, but was normal again now. I reworked the colon area several times until it felt less sensitive. The lymph around the ankles were still causing sensitivity so I applied extra gentle work to them with yet more gliding and draining movements. On finishing the treatment the ankles and feet were visibly less swollen. I recommended that her husband collected her from her next treatment, and that if he came 15 minutes before the end I would show him the opening movements, the gentle lymph drainage movements around the ankle and the closing movements. She thought this was a fantastic idea. I felt it would be a great home maintenance treatment between my sessions and suggested that he apply the technique every other day, preferably before bedtime so that she did not have to stand again directly afterwards.

At the next session she reported an increase in urination, but that this was probably due to my advice to increase her water intake! Her ankles were much less swollen than at the start of the previous treatment and she also reported a great improvement to the swelling of her hands. She was very positive about the results so far.

There were very few sensitive areas during the treatment, with only the lymph and lumbar vertebrae (spine, lumbar 3/4/5) still sensitive. When I asked about her lower back she said it felt fine but that she had been gardening several times during the week. I thought that she enjoyed her work too much to stop because of sensitive reactions to the spinal reflexes, so I just mentioned that she should be aware of her posture and ease up if she felt any pain. We also joked about the baby repositioning itself due to her many gardening positions and she commented that she would probably give birth in the garden!

Her husband arrived early so that I could demonstrate the movements I had previously discussed with her. I took one foot to demonstrate the opening movements while he took the other and followed. I also showed him some lymph work around the ankle and upper lymph work between the toes. We finished with the closing movements. I then watched while he did the movements. I was amazed at how quickly he picked them up. I suggested that he practise this routine on his wife every other day.

When I saw the client the following week she reported the amazing effect of her husband's treatment. When I examined the feet it was absolutely true – there was virtually no swelling or discomfort. I suggested that her husband might wish to consider a change of career!

The treatment did not result in any major areas of sensitivity, apart from the lymph areas, and even here it was much reduced. There was also slight sensitivity around the sciatic reflex areas (right foot). On working the diaphragm she reported a large kick from the baby!

I treated this client three more times and suggested she return if any new problems arose. Her husband had kept up the treatments and she was much better.

Some time later she wrote with news of the birth of a healthy baby boy, and that the birth had been painful but quick! She also mentioned that her husband was still giving her the 'mini' treatments and that as a thank you she was going to book a reflexology treatment for him.

At this point it is worth mentioning that I have treated many pregnant woman as well as women who are trying to conceive or undergoing infertility treatment (IVF). I have never had any problems or complications while treating these clients.

There are several schools of thought about treating infertility and pregnant women. It is of great value for the qualified reflexologist to attend specialist workshops or seminars on these subjects to expand their knowledge and confidence in treating clients with these conditions. My own advice is that if the client is unsure about the reflexology treatment, is on medication or has had complications with a past pregnancy, then they should check with their consultant or doctor before receiving a treatment. Likewise if you do not feel confident administering a treatment, then you should refer the client to a practitioner with specialist skill or knowledge in this area. My belief is that if you treat with love and care you will be very unlikely to cause harm. It is also true that some practitioners have very good results using extremely light pressure – so remember there is never one way to approach the treatment, you must rely on the combination of your reflexology skills and your intuition.

CHAPTER 31

Thoughts on the reflexology treatment

I hope that the case studies have helped to demonstrate the individual treatment approach required for each client. It is always important to remember that a disease or physical problem is a condition of the whole person. If a client refuses or is unable to deal with difficult situations then this can bring on many associated problems. If we are able to treat the client during these times of difficulty then we are more able to help the client to intervene and fight against the onset of a particular disease or condition. It is also worth remembering that some clients' presenting conditions or inability to deal with situations comes not from recent events, but from events in the past. These conditions could be viewed as an imbalance in their life force or constitution.

Most of us are ultimately responsible for our own conditions, which can usually be improved with certain lifestyle and environmental changes, given the willingness of the client to participate in the treatment process. As therapists we also participate in the healing process by enabling a client to help take responsibility for their own health and by stimulating the body's own corrective healing potential.

The more the client is aware of themselves the quicker and more fulfilling the treatment process will be. It is important for both client and practitioner to remain in contact with the purpose of the treatment and to focus on the potential benefits.

Believe it or not there is a disadvantage to the holistic approach – the length of the treatment period. Many clients want a speedy treatment, a quick fix with an immediate solution to their condition. The client must have patience with the treatment process. Thankfully the advantages far outweigh the disadvantages, and if we can influence the overall deep health of the client and enable them to move on with their life, the time invested by both parties will reap great benefits. The changes to a client's health are not only in the symptoms but also in the overall approach to their own mental, spiritual and emotional life. They can, quite literally become a 'whole' person.

CHAPTER 32

Coursework, case studies and written examination preparation

COURSEWORK

When presenting a coursework folder it is important to remember that it is a reflection of your attitude and commitment towards reflexology. Spend time organising the coursework so that it shows your full potential. The main points to bear in mind are:

1. Put your name on the front of the folder.

2. Include an index as a first page – this should explain where everything is in the file.

3. Make sure every page can be read by turning over the pages. Do not bundle several pages together in a plastic wallet.

4. Include your rough notes and jottings – these do not have to be neatly written. It is evidence of your own follow-up work.

5. Include any rough diagrams and notes you have made of the reflexology sequence – these show you have been practising.

6. Include any answers to tasks and test sheets – this shows evidence of study.

7. Include a list of books and articles read or referred to during your studies – this shows evidence of self-study and motivation.

8. Make sure the file is organised – for example by subject order or date order. This shows evidence of preparation and professionalism.

9. If you have to hand in a course file for inspection, make sure you do so on time.

Do not worry if your notes are handwritten – as long as they are clear.

 Task 80 • Check your coursework folder, if you have one, and ensure that it is well organised, using the above for guidance.

CASE STUDIES

When compiling a folder of consultations and treatments given as part of your studies it is important to have them in a logical order:

1. Include a front index page indicating treatments given – an example is shown below.

2. Organise the file with a section for each client treated, in date order.

3. Use codes instead of names and addresses to preserve client's anonymity. For example, client A, client B etc. A confidential list of the names and addresses as they relate to the codes should be kept.

Example front page index sheet for client treatment file:

Client	Original presenting condition/reason for treatment	Total number of treatments	Date of first and last treatment	Page number in file
Mr A	General relaxation	10	1/3/2002–23/6/2002	2–15
Mr B	Lumbar back pain	12	1/5/2002–13/8/2002	16–30
Miss C	Exhaustion/tired all the time	10	1/6/2002–31/8/2002	31–43
Mr D	General relaxation	15	1/7/2002–30/8/2002	44–60
Mrs B	Migraine	5	6/3/2002–12/5/2002	61–66
TOTAL		52	1/3/2002–31/8/2002	

This is just an example, you may approach the index page in a different way and show different information – it is the general approach that is important.

 Task 81 • Check your case history/client treatment folder, if you have one, and ensure that it is well organised, using the above for guidance

PREPARING FOR WRITTEN EXAMINATIONS

Not many people enjoy sitting a written examination, but there are some things that you can do to make it less traumatic:

1. **Plan in advance.** You will know the date of a final written exam well in advance. This gives you time to prepare. Set out a revision timetable and stick to it.

2. **Test yourself.** After you have revised a particular topic test yourself with questions and see how you do.

   Get together in a small group if possible – you can then help each other.

3. **Sit a pretend exam.** Try to get hold of a past exam paper and make yourself do it in the time allowed. If you can't get a paper make one up with questions you think might appear.

4. **Final two weeks.** In the final two weeks before an exam draw up a final revision plan, allocating time to particular topics. This should be on a rotational basis over five days – so that you can repeat it twice before the exam day.

5. **On the exam day.** Don't panic! Arrive in plenty of time. Look through the paper first to get a feel for all the questions.

   Start with the questions you feel best able to answer – this will then give you confidence for the others.

   Don't get stuck! Don't spend a lot of time on one difficult question when you could be answering three others instead.

   Be strict with your time. Make sure you allow enough time to answer each question – keep an eye on the clock.

   If you feel overwhelmed by the situation take two minutes out – sit and take deep breaths, clear your mind, and then begin again.

6. **The final minutes . . .** Check your name is on the exam paper and that you have followed all the administrative instructions. Check that all your answers are included and that no part of the answer paper has gone missing.

   Congratulate yourself on a job well done!

Chapter 33 contains a useful summary of all tasks contained in this book, which can be used as part of your revision planning.

 Task 82 • **Use the revision guide chapter to test your reflexology knowledge.**

Revision guide

Throughout this book there have been tasks to help reinforce the information given in the chapters. Many of the tasks are based on possible examination type questions (although this will vary depending on which exam you are taking).

If you are revising for a final written examination it will be helpful to test yourself using some of the tasks without referring back to the answers within the text. Here is a selection of the tasks for you to answer. The chapters where you will find the answers are given next to each task so that you can check your answers afterwards.

If you are using this book for self-study it would still be useful to test yourself to see how much information you have remembered.

Good luck!

Task Note: this is a selection of the tasks featured in the book – the numbers do not refer to the actual task numbers within the book.	Chapter containing the answer
1. List four actual reactions that a client may have after receiving a reflexology treatment.	4
2. Briefly describe the major contributions made to reflexology by the following people: a) Dr William Fitzgerald b) Dr Joe Shelby Riley c) Hanne Marquardt	5
3. a) Describe the important principal established by Sir Charles Sherrington (1861–1952) in his work *The Integrative Action of the Nervous System* which later went on to win him the Nobel prize. b) Who is widely regarded as having introduced reflexology into the United Kingdom? c) Approximately when did this take place?	5

Task			Chapter containing the answer
4.	a)	Give two experiences/sources of knowledge that may have influenced Dr William Fitzgerald in his development of zone therapy.	5
	b)	Name three influences that are affecting the development of our therapy today.	
5.	a)	Give two ways in which the Eastern method of reflexology (e.g. Chinese, Rwo Shur) differs from that practised in the West.	
	b)	Name two practices that are related to or that developed from reflexology but which are regarded in the UK as separate therapies.	5
6.	a)	On a template of the right foot, using your preferred reflex chart, draw in the location of the following six reflexes and label each one:	6
		Adrenals Hip Shoulder	
		Bladder Pituitary Sinuses	
	b)	Name two reflexes that may be accessed on the dorsal surface of the foot as well as the more normal position on the plantar surface.	
7.	a)	Give two explanations for the fact that there are many different charts, with reflexes in different locations.	6
	b)	Briefly describe zone theory.	
	c)	How is the arrangement of zones on the big toes different from the rest of the foot.	
	d)	Why do reflexologists often work the kidneys to help an eye disorder.	
8.	a)	What is a cross reflex (also known as a referral area)?	6
	b)	Give four examples of cross reflexes.	
	c)	Give two reasons why you might use a cross reflex.	

Task	Chapter
Note: this is a selection of the tasks featured in the book – the numbers do not refer to the actual task numbers within the book.	containing the answer
9. a) On a right foot template draw in and label the lateral/ transverse zones of the feet on both plantar and dorsal aspects. b) On a left foot template draw in and label the longitudinal zones.	6
10. Does it make any difference which foot is used to start the treatment. State why you begin on your chosen foot.	7
11. a) Describe four situations in which you might lighten your normal pressure. b) Reflexologists make observations and assessments from the feel of the foot. List six different sensations that may be felt by the therapist through touch during the course of a treatment or several treatments.	7
12. Give five possible reasons why a particular reflex might be sensitive or out of balance.	7
13. Many practitioners give extra attention to reflex areas felt to be out of balance. Describe three ways in which you might include such work in your treatment session.	7
14. a) What do you understand is meant by the term contraindication? b) Name two conditions that some practitioners consider to be major contraindications to reflexology treatment.	8
15. a) Name two conditions that may indicate caution is required during treatment; give the condition and reason for caution in each case. b) Give two indications that show a client may be having a hypersensitive response during treatment.	8

Task		Chapter containing the answer
16. a)	Describe the condition commonly known as athlete's foot. Give a possible cause of such a condition.	9
b)	What is the conventional treatment for athlete's foot?	
17. a)	i) Describe the condition known as a 'bunion'.	9
	ii) Give two possible causes of such a condition.	
b)	i) What is a skin callous?	
	ii) Give two causes of such a condition.	
c)	Describe a possible treatment for:	
	i) a bunion	
	ii) a callous.	
18. a)	Name four conditions of the feet that could result from diabetes mellitus.	9
b)	i) State which of the following foot conditions are infectious. Corns Verrucae Eczema	
	ii) What precaution can be taken by the reflexologist to prevent contraction of the infection?	
c)	Name two conditions affecting the toenail, and a possible cause for each.	
19. a)	What important function do the calf muscles perform in relation to the circulation in the foot	9
b)	Name three conditions that may involve a disorder of the circulation of the feet.	
20. a)	Name two of the main weight-bearing bones in the foot.	9
b)	What are the two main functions of the foot?	
c)	To which bone and muscles is the Achilles tendon attached?	

Task	Chapter
Note: this is a selection of the tasks featured in the book – the numbers do not refer to the actual task numbers within the book.	containing the answer

21.	a) How many bones are there in each foot?	9
	b) Give two functions of the arches of the foot?	
	c) Name four of the bones that form the tarsus.	
	d) i) What are sesamoid bones?	
	ii) Where are they found in the foot?	
	iii) What are their function?	
22.	a) Name six common disorders of the feet.	9
	b) State two ways in which the skin on the sole of the foot is different from that elsewhere on the body.	
23.	a) Give two reasons why a client may prefer to have a hand reflexology treatment.	10
	b) Give three reasons why you might give a hand reflexology treatment instead of a foot reflexology treatment.	
	c) Give two reasons why the use of some hand reflexology (as opposed to a full treatment) might be appropriate.	
24.	a) Describe three possible positions for client and practitioner to receive a hand reflexology treatment.	10
	b) Describe three ways in which working on the hands differs from the feet.	
25.	a) List four diseases or conditions that can be found on the hands.	10
	b) What is carpal tunnel syndrome and what are the symptoms?	
26.	When seeing a client for the first time it is important to take an initial consultation. List what you consider to be five important questions that should be asked and recorded before the first treatment begins.	11

Task	Chapter containing the answer
27. a) Give four reasons why it is important to keep a record of each treatment given to a client. b) Name what you consider to be four of the most important items to include when completing your record of a treatment session.	11
28. Describe two ways in which you would ensure that client records remained confidential.	11
29. As reflexologists, apart from looking at the feet, we should observe our clients for other clues to their general condition and state of well being. List four of the clues we could look for.	12
30. As reflexologists we may look for indicators to a client's health by observing the condition of the feet or noting the differences between the feet. a) List eight of these indicators that may be present on a visual examination of a client's feet. b) Give two possible assessments that could be made from the observation that your client has very wet, perspiring feet.	12
31. Give a possible problem each of the following conditions might indicate in the body: a) Ingrowing toenail b) Fallen longitudinal arch c) Bunion.	12
32. List three basic ways a reflexologist assesses the condition and treatment needs of a client.	12
33. List four points you would make to a new or prospective client when describing to them what to expect during a treatment session.	14

Task	Chapter
Note: this is a selection of the tasks featured in the book – the numbers do not refer to the actual task numbers within the book.	containing the answer

34. a) Detail two responses you could give if a client asked, 'Why does that point hurt?' — 14

   b) Describe four points you would make to a client when giving your aftercare advice at the end of a treatment.

35. a) Explain to a client two advantages and two disadvantages of self-treatment. — 14

   b) Give a possible reason behind each of the statements listed below:

   i) I always give my clients a card with the date and time of their next treatment.

   ii) I like to help clients on and off the treatment chair or couch.

36. a) List four common reactions a client may experience after a reflexology treatment.

   b) Give three possible reasons why a client may have a reaction after treatment. — 14

37. Name four other complementary therapies that might help a client with back pain. Give a brief description of each therapy. — 15

38. a) Give two reasons why you might consider referring a client to another complementary health practitioner, apart from a reflexologist. — 15

   b) Compile a list of four questions that, in your opinion, a prospective client should ask any complementary practitioner to establish their credentials and suitability before deciding upon treatment.

39. State two circumstances when you would ask a client to consult their GP or other medical professional. — 15

Task	Chapter containing the answer

40. A client suffering from cystitis comes for treatment.　16

    a)　i) Describe this condition.

        ii) Give two possible causes or triggers.

    b)　Name the key reflex area and two other areas that could be given particular attention to help ease the complaint, and give a reason for each.

41. A client suffering from insomnia comes for treatment.　16

    a)　i) Describe this condition.

    b)　ii) Give two possible causes or triggers.

    b)　Name the key reflex area and two other areas that could be given particular attention to help ease the complaint, and give a reason for each.

42. a)　Give a one or two sentence general definition of 'stress'.　18

    b)　List four factors that may cause or contribute towards stress.

    c)　List what you consider to be two of the most important reflex areas to treat stress. Give your reason in each case.

43. a)　Name two lifestyle factors that could cause, trigger or predispose someone to each of the following conditions:　18

        i) Arteriosclerosis

        ii) Diabetes mellitus

        iii) Cervical cancer

        iv) Depression

        v) Varicose veins.

    b)　A client presents with persistent headaches. The doctor finds nothing medically wrong. Give five possible environmental or lifestyle factors that may be contributing to the condition, and give a brief reason for each.

Task	Chapter containing the answer
Note: this is a selection of the tasks featured in the book – the numbers do not refer to the actual task numbers within the book.	
44. a) Define hypertension in one or two sentences	18
b) Name four lifestyle factors that may alter normal blood pressure.	
c) Give four reasons why exercise is important for good health.	
45. a) Give an example of how, in your opinion, mental attitude/emotions can affect the physical health of the body.	19
b) Mention five points that are distinguishing features of the holistic approach to health.	
46. a) A visit to the doctor can result in symptoms of an illness being alleviated, but often the patient still does not feel better. From a holistic perspective, give one reason why this might be so.	19
b) What might be a benefit of treating the mother of a child who has been brought to you for treatment?	
c) Give two ways in which your listening skills could benefit your client.	
47. a) Briefly explain the concept of the healing crisis.	19
b) List three self-help activities or methods that might help a client to let go of negative mental patterns and develop a more positive outlook on life.	
48. a) Describe what you understand by the subtle body.	20
b) List four effects that might be experienced by a reflexologist or a client during a treatment that could be due to an exchange of subtle energy.	
c) Name two ways in which we receive/absorb the lifeforce or vital energy.	

Task			Chapter containing the answer
49.	a)	List four mental or physical factors that could impede the flow of life energies through the body.	20
	b)	list four indications that could be present on the feet if a client is low in 'vital' energy.	
50.		Name four therapies that work with energies that flow through the body.	20
51.	a)	Give four reasons why the body needs food.	21
	b)	Name four of the basic nutritional components of a balanced diet.	
	c)	Give two reasons why fibre is important in the diet.	
	d)	List two minerals that are important for bone growth and repair.	
52.	a)	Give two reasons why the body needs vitamin A.	21
	b)	Name two food sources that contain vitamin A	
	c)	Name two types of food that contain iron.	
	d)	What effect would iron deficiency have on the body.	
53.	a)	List what you consider to be six important considerations when designing and equipping a treatment room.	22
	b)	Give two reasons why hygiene in your practice is important.	
54.		List what you consider to be four important factors in the way practitioners present themselves. Give your reason in each case.	22
55.	a)	What are two of the main reasons for establishing a Code of Ethics for reflexologists?	23
	b)	Name three types of misconduct, which could result in disciplinary procedure against a member.	
	c)	Give three reasons why you might refuse to treat a client.	

Task	Chapter containing the answer
Note: this is a selection of the tasks featured in the book – the numbers do not refer to the actual task numbers within the book.	

56.	a)	Why should practitioners be aware of local and national support systems?	23
	b)	How might you find out about the existence of organisation and support networks? Give three sources.	
57.	a)	Give three advantages and three disadvantages of running a clinic from home.	24
	b)	Give two advantages and two disadvantages of working from a group complementary clinic.	
58.	a)	Give three advantages and three disadvantages of been self-employed.	24
	b)	Give three advantages and three disadvantages of carrying out home visits to clients.	
59.	a)	In any advertising what do you consider to be the three most important general principles? Give a reason in each case.	25
	b)	List four items of business stationery that you would consider to be important for the running of your business.	
	c)	What, in your opinion, are three of the most useful pieces of information to include on any publicity information?	
60.	a)	Give one advantage and one disadvantage of newspaper advertising.	25
	b)	Apart from the above, give four other marketing methods for promoting yourself as a reflexologist.	
61.	a)	i) What do you understand by the term professional negligence?	26
		ii) State two ways in which can you safeguard yourself from possible claims of professional negligence.	
	b)	i) What is the main provision of the Trade Descriptions Act 1968?	
		ii) Explain the importance of this to practitioners.	

Task	Chapter containing the answer
62. The law lists prohibited functions, which are certain specified functions within the field of medicine that unqualified persons are forbidden to perform. State two of these prohibited functions.	26
63. a) What do you understand by the term Local Authority Licence or Special Treatment Licence in relation to the practice of reflexology? b) Describe how you would establish whether a local authority had licence requirements.	26

64. a) What do you understand by the following terms:
  i) National Insurance
  ii) Tax allowance?
b) What information would a notice of coding give you?
	27

65. a) Give two possible tax effects of using a room in your home exclusively for business. b) What information does a bank statement give you? c) As a self-employed person you are required to keep certain records for accounting purposes. Give three of the categories of information that must be kept.	27

66. What do you understand by the following terms:
  i) VAT
  ii) Net profit?
	27

67. a) What are the names of the two essential types of insurance a practitioner should have before treating the public? Explain the purpose of each. b) Besides the above, name two other types of insurance that may be needed by a reflexologist.	28

Task	Chapter
Note: this is a selection of the tasks featured in the book – the numbers do not refer to the actual task numbers within the book.	**containing the answer**

CHAPTER 34

Care for the therapist

You may have heard the phrase 'practitioner burn out' being used to describe those practitioners who feel that they have just had enough of their work and are too exhausted to treat any more clients or even to treat one more ever again!

It may seem a little early for you to think about burn out – you may feel that it is a problem that affects other people – but it is something that all practitioners need to be aware of as the more clients we begin to treat, the more it tends to creep up on us, without much warning. Part of the problem is that we are all natural helpers, otherwise we would not be attracted to the caring professions in the first place. This often means we have a deep sense of wanting to help and care for others and to help them.

This driving force means we can neglect our well-being for the sake of others. We will see one more client when we really have seen enough for the day. We will go that extra distance for a home visit, even if it means rushing around for the rest of the day to get back on schedule. We will spend extra time on a treatment even if our hands and back begin to ache. We will spend time thinking about certain client's problems long after the treatment session has ended and begin to get too emotionally involved, and so on . . .

The effects of burn out are cumulative. We may not notice it after each incident but the constant build-up will eventually cause us concern. It is for this reason that you need to think of a strategy for helping yourself as well as helping others. This is not selfish behaviour, for you cannot help your clients to help themselves unless you are in a fit state to administer the treatment.

Here are some strategies for you to think about and, more importantly, put into practise from day one. Don't wait until it is too late.

1. Be gentle with yourself

    Remind yourself that you are an enabler NOT a magician. You cannot be expected to be the instant 'quick fix' solution for your clients. The equation does not read:

    $$\frac{\text{Your maximum effort}}{\text{Their spare time}} = \text{their quick recovery}$$

but rather

$$\frac{\text{Your treatment} \times \text{Your encouragement}}{\text{Their involvement in the treatment}} = \text{their ability to change and improve}$$

It is not always the case that a client will improve with treatments, but do not take this as a sign of your own failure or inadequacy. Many factors are involved, including the client's own perception of their illness and their own ideas about when and how they will get better. Such ideas are definitely beyond your control. Accept this and move on.

2. Find a hermit spot – use it daily

    Always set aside some time for yourself during each day, even if only for ten minutes. Find somewhere quiet and try to clear your head of all thoughts. This is not an easy task, but when random thoughts do fly into your head try to imagine them flying out again! The very act of seeking stillness will help to counteract the stress of the day.

3. Give support, encouragement and praise. Learn to accept it in return

    Always try to give support and praise to others, not just to your clients but to people in the rest of your life. The very act of encouragement makes both parties feel good about themselves. It is also important to accept praise in return. You are allowed to feel you have achieved, and can be rewarded by others. Your sense of well-being will be much increased.

4. Remember that in the light of all the pain that we see, we are bound to feel helpless at times

    Admit it without shame. Caring and being there are sometimes more important than doing. Pain is part of life.

5. Change your routine and your tasks when you can

    Try to vary your work hours. Do your routine tasks at different times of the day, if possible. This will help keep the boredom at bay. Vary your approaches to the treatment with different clients, try new techniques. Be a resource to yourself. Get creative – try new approaches. Be an artist as well as a technician.

6. Learn to recognise the difference between complaining that relieves and complaining that reinforces negative stress and negative thought patterns

    Learn to protect yourself from negative thoughts and emotions when expressed by clients. They are entitled to their negative thought patterns, and indeed this is sometimes part of the treatment process, but do not allow this to penentrate your own being. On the way home, or when finishing work, focus on a good thing that has happened during the day.

7. Use your colleagues regularly as a source of support, assurance and redirection

    Talk to other therapists who understand your work. Share your fun moments as well as your concerns. Help each other with ideas and swap treatments.

8. Avoid shop talk during breaks and when socialising

    Mix with others who are not in the therapy business. Get a different angle on life. Try different interests and hobbys and don't always get dragged into being the 'on-hand therapist encylopedia'. If you are worried about too many therapy questions, don't mention that you're a therapist!

9. Say 'I choose' rather than 'I should'

    Don't punish yourself with too many rules and regulations. Accept that things have to be done and do them. Make choices where you can.

10. If you never say no – what is your 'yes' worth?

    Never be afraid to say no. Often when we say 'I'll think about it' or 'I'm not sure' we really mean *no* – but just can't say it! Practise in front of a mirror if you have a saying *no* problem. Above all else remember that saying yes all the time does not mean instant approval and respect from everyone.

11. Aloofness and indifference are far more harmful than admitting an inability to do or know more

    Don't be afraid to admit the limits of your knowledge. Never try to cover up with excuses or a superior attitude, this will just antagonise others and lose the respect you are working so hard to gain. People respect honesty above all else.

12. Take up something for yourself

    Find another interest, for example meditation, sport, creative visualisation, self-hypnosis, good diet, Bach flower remedies, homoeopathy, Alexandra Technique, essential oils, affirmations.

13. Laugh and play

    Make sure you have a really good time at least once a week. Do something to make you laugh and play.

Further study and reflexology training

I would like to recommend the following for further study:

James, Andrew, 1998. *Hands on Reflexology, training video*. www.handsonreflexology.com

Page, Dr Christine, 1992 *Frontiers of Health*. C. W. Daniel, London. ISBN 0852073402

Excellent for learning more about the holistic approach to health.

Grinberg, Avi, 1993. *Reflexology foot analysis*. Samiel Weiser Inc., USA. ISBN 0877287805

An interesting and well-thought-out approach to reflexology.

Ingham, Eunice, 1984. *The original works of Eunice D. Ingham – stories the feet can tell and stories the feet have told through reflexology*. Ingham Publishing Inc., Florida. ISBN 0961180439

An insight into the mind and technique of an early pioneer of reflexology.

British Medical Association, 1992, *The Complete Family Health Encyclopaedia*. Dorling Kindersley, London. ISBN 0863184383

An excellent reference book for a wide range of medical conditions, their causes and possible treatment.

Copeland, Glen, D. P. M., 1991. *The foot book*. John Wiley & Sons, New York. ISBN 0471199176

Advice, help and information on foot-related conditions.

FOR REFLEXOLOGY TRAINING

For accredited practitioner level training, to become a member of the Association of Reflexologists or for an AoR practitioner in your area write for details to:

The Association of Reflexologists

27 Old Gloucester Street

London WC1N 3XX

www.aor.org.uk

For practitioner training with Andrew James visit

www.handsonreflexology.com

where you will find further information and be able to download clips from the training video.

Index

Index

Index

263